Imaging for Surgical Disease

Editors

Raphael Sun, MD
General Surgery Resident
Department of Surgery
University of Iowa Hospitals and Clinics
Iowa City, Iowa

David Ring, MD
General Surgery Resident
Department of Surgery
University of Iowa Hospitals and Clinics
Iowa City, Iowa

Steven Sauk, MD
Vascular and Interventional Radiology Fellow
Mallinckrodt Institute of Radiology
Washington University in St. Louis
St. Louis, Missouri

Hui Sen Chong, MD
Assistant Professor
Department of Surgery
University of Iowa Hospitals and Clinics
Iowa City, Iowa

Wolters Kluwer | Lippincott Williams & Wilkins
Health
Philadelphia · Baltimore · New York · London
Buenos Aires · Hong Kong · Sydney · Tokyo

Acquisitions Editor: Keith Donnellan
Product Manager: Brendan Huffman
Production Manager: Priscilla Crater
Senior Manufacturing Manager: Beth Welsh
Marketing Manager: Lisa Lawrence
Design Coordinator: Teresa Mallon
Production Service: Aptara, Inc.

Printed in China

Library of Congress Cataloging-in-Publication Data

Imaging for surgical disease / editors, Raphael Sun, David Ring, Steven Sauk, Hui Sen Chong.
    pages ; cm
    Includes bibliographical references.
    ISBN 978-1-4511-8638-3 (paperback)
    I. Sun, Raphael, editor. II. Ring, David, active 2013, editor.
III. Sauk, Steven, editor. IV. Chong, Hui Sen, editor.
    [DNLM: 1. Radiography. 2. Surgical Procedures, Operative. WN 200]
    RC78.7.T6
    616.07′572—dc23
                                                                2013018376

Care has been taken to confirm the accuracy of the information presented and to describe generally accepted practices. However, the authors, editors, and publisher are not responsible for errors or omissions or for any consequences from application of the information in this book and make no warranty, expressed or implied, with respect to the currency, completeness, or accuracy of the contents of the publication. Application of the information in a particular situation remains the professional responsibility of the practitioner.

The authors, editors, and publisher have exerted every effort to ensure that drug selection and dosage set forth in this text are in accordance with current recommendations and practice at the time of publication. However, in view of ongoing research, changes in government regulations, and the constant flow of information relating to drug therapy and drug reactions, the reader is urged to check the package insert for each drug for any change in indications and dosage and for added warnings and precautions. This is particularly important when the recommended agent is a new or infrequently employed drug.

Some drugs and medical devices presented in the publication have Food and Drug Administration (FDA) clearance for limited use in restricted research settings. It is the responsibility of the health care provider to ascertain the FDA status of each drug or device planned for use in their clinical practice.

To purchase additional copies of this book, call our customer service department at (800) 638-3030 or fax orders to (301) 223-2320. International customers should call (301) 223-2300.

Visit Lippincott Williams & Wilkins on the Internet: at LWW.com. Lippincott Williams & Wilkins customer service representatives are available from 8:30 am to 6 pm, EST.

CCS0913

Dedications

To my mother and father who sacrificed everything to get me to where I am today. To my best friends, you are my brothers, and to Li, for your unconditional love.

A special thanks to Dr. Scott-Conner. Your mentorship throughout this process helped make this wonderful book possible.

—Raphael Sun

For my beautiful wife and daughter, the most supportive mom and brothers anyone could ask for, and my dad who I miss dearly—I love you all.

—David Ring

To my family—Mom, Dad, Jenny, and Kevin—for their unparalleled love and support, and to Jane, for making me the luckiest man in the world.

—Steven Sauk

To my partner Kent and to my family Yew Kiang, Sew Ying, Tsen Tze, Hui Ming, and Tsen Yi for their never-ending support.

—Hui Sen Chong

Contributors

Simon Roh, MD
Radiology Resident
Department of Radiology
University of Iowa Hospitals
  and Clinics
Iowa City, Iowa

Melhem Sharafuddin, MD
Clinical Associate Professor
Department of Surgery
University of Iowa Hospitals
  and Clinics
Iowa City, Iowa

Maheen Rajput, MD
Clinical Assistant Professor
Department of Radiology
University of Iowa Hospitals
  and Clinics
Iowa City, Iowa

Muneera Kapadia, MD
Clinical Assistant Professor
Department of Surgery
University of Iowa Hospitals
  and Clinics
Iowa City, Iowa

Michele Lilienthal, RN, MA, CEN
Trauma Program Manager
Department of Surgery
University of Iowa Hospitals
  and Clinics
Iowa City, Iowa

Hisakazu Hoshi, MD
Clinical Associate Professor
Department of Surgery
University of Iowa Hospitals
  and Clinics
Iowa City, Iowa

James Mezhir, MD
Assistant Professor
Department of Surgery
University of Iowa Hospitals
  and Clinics
Iowa City, Iowa

Preface

General surgery deals with all areas of the human body. Although history and physical examination still provide the foundation of diagnosis, radiologic imaging is a part of the patient evaluation in modern practice. Most patients who undergo an operation have some sort of radiologic imaging. One common example is acute appendicitis. This disease used to be a clinical diagnosis. Barium enemas, and later ultrasound, were introduced to confirm or exclude the diagnosis in the difficult cases. These modalities have now been superseded by CT of the abdomen. This radiologic test has almost become a standard of practice for patients who present with right lower quadrant pain.

Surgery residency training includes the expectation that residents will be able to use radiographic imaging to help confirm diagnosis and to plan treatment options, yet residents do not receive formal training in radiology. Residents are often expected to see a patient, take the history and physical examination and order a type of imaging that will help decide the treatment plan. However, we residents find it difficult to look at images without any background knowledge or training. Many times residents will look at the images, read the radiologist's report, and then look once again at the images to see what the radiologist was referring to. At the end of the process, the surgical resident still may not be able to identify the positive finding on the images.

Residency training is busy and filled with textbook readings, yearly ABSITE reviews, extracurricular research, journal articles and presentations. Little time is dedicated to learning how to read radiology images.

This book, *Imaging for Surgical Diseases*, provides a tool and a simple guide for residents to be able to identify common surgical diseases. Each section of the book is dedicated to one specific disease process. In each section, there are radiology images demonstrating positive findings. These images are clearly labeled to highlight the area of interest and also the surrounding anatomy for reference points. Each section contains information on both the surgical and radiologic aspects of the disease. The surgery part contains a basic summary including clinical signs and symptoms. The radiology part specifies helpful hints that pertain to the certain disease.

This book is sized to fit conveniently in a resident's white coat pocket. There have been many radiology books that teach basic radiology and there are even textbooks published that are meant for surgeons in clinical practice. However, there are no books so far that are personalized and simplified for the surgical resident or medical student.

Our textbook is written by practicing surgeons who have clinical experience. Our approach is to use radiology to help confirm the diagnosis. This style of practice fits the objectives and the curriculum of general surgery residency. Our text concentrates on the most common radiology images that surgery residents order every day, rather than including the esoteric. Instead of paragraph format, the information is presented in bullet and outline format, making it brief and concise. This allows a resident to quickly refer to the handbook as a practical guide as opposed to a reference textbook.

The goal of this book is simple. It is intended to be a compact handbook that will help residents become familiar with radiology imaging that is related to the surgical patient. It also will allow the resident to learn which diagnostic imaging is appropriate for any given patient and how it should be ordered. This book is intended to help train surgical residents to become independent practicing clinicians.

Contents

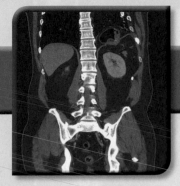

Introduction: Radiology Overview

Chest Plain Films

Reading plain films requires a systematic approach to ensure that no pathologies are missed. Various different approaches exist and a clinician needs to find a method that works best for him/her. A method that has been used widely will be reviewed here. Reading a chest film can be done using the ABCDs.

Airway. One needs to look at the airways to make sure there are no strictures, masses, or other foreign bodies which may be obstructing the air passage. The trachea is noted in the center of the chest plain film as a linear, vertical lucency starting from the thyroid down to the carina which leads to the left and right main bronchi. The right main bronchus divides into three lobar bronchi while left main bronchus divides into two lobar bronchi. Lobar bronchi divide into multiple tertiary bronchi. Following the lucency up to the level of the main bronchi will be possible with properly developed chest plain film.

Bones/**B**reast shadow. Reviewing the bones is crucial to make sure nothing is missed. Start at the top and work your way down. Make sure no spinal deformities, clavicle/scapular/rib fractures are present. Breast shadow can create a diffuse haziness along the inferior aspect of the lung fields. Be sure to not mistake the increased opacity of the lower lung fields for a pulmonary process such as atelectasis or infiltrate.

Cardiac/**C**ostophrenic angle. A careful inspection of the heart size and borders is mandatory. The right atrium forms the right border of cardiac silhouette. Right ventricle forms the inferior border of the heart against the diaphragm. Left ventricle forms the apex of the heart. Left atrium forms the left upper border of the heart. The aortic knob forms a bulge toward the upper aspect of the heart shadow. The ratio of heart width to thoracic cavity should be less than 0.55 on PA view. Costophrenic angles should have a clear and acute angle. Any blunting of this angle indicates an effusion.

Diaphragm. Carefully inspect beneath the diaphragm to make sure there is no free air. Free air will be indicated by areas of lucency immediately underneath the diaphragm. Do not mistake gastric bubble as free air. Upon maximum inspiration, the medial borders of the diaphragm should have a relatively flattened appearance.

Edges/**E**xtrathoracic tissues. Inspect the lung apices for fibrosis or pneumothorax. In pneumothorax, a fine line indicating the edge of the lung will be present. Pulmonary vasculature will be absent peripheral to the lung edge. Do not mistake skin folds or other extrathoracic tissues for pleural edge.

Fields. The lung fields should be clear with pulmonary vasculature most prominent around the hila. Any increase in opacity of the lung fields should lead to suspicion of acute pulmonary processes such as pneumonia, atelectasis, effusion, etc.

Abdomen Plain Films

Abdominal plain films are obtained for suspicion of acute abdominal processes such as bowel obstruction, perforation, or other pathologies which may lead to abdominal pain. Careful inspection of the bowel loops are indicated when reading an abdominal plain film. In most cases, small bowel does not contain any visible gas. Significant amounts of gas within small bowel loops should lead one to think of an obstructive process especially if air–fluid levels are present. Adynamic ileus will also result in air–fluid levels within the small bowel as well. Differentiating between the two is difficult on a plain film, however, in ileus, the large bowel is more likely to be distended as well. Multiple air–fluid levels arranged in a stepladder-like appearance indicate that the obstruction is distal.

Perforation of the bowels will result in free air. In an upright abdominal plain film, the spaces immediately beneath the diaphragm should be carefully inspected for any lucency which may indicate free air. In questionable cases, a left lateral decubitus should be obtained which will show air bubbles along the right peritoneum. A right lateral decubitus film is not advised as air bubbles accumulating along the left peritoneum may be confused with gastric bubble.

The biliary tract should be carefully inspected for suspicion of free air within the bile ducts which may be indicated by free air within the ducts.

Chronic pancreatitis may show calcification along the area occupied by the pancreas. Acute pancreatitis will not be visible on a plain film.

Pelvis Plain Films

Pelvic plain films are usually obtained in the setting of trauma. A careful inspection of the pelvis is mandatory. One should follow along the edges of the pelvis to look for disruption of the cortical surfaces. Any disruption or incongruity of the edges should lead one to suspect a pelvic fracture. The femoral head and proximal shaft, as well as the acetabulum, should be closely inspected for signs of fracture. Paying attention to the pelvic symmetry will also reveal any signs for pelvic disruption.

CT: Chest

CT of the chest is performed to better delineate the mediastinal and pulmonary structures. Start by looking at the lungs in the lung window to see if any apical pneumothorax exists. Pneumothorax is shown by black lucency. Scroll down the lung fields to check for other pathologies. Pneumonia or pleural effusions will be noted by increased opacities.

Next, move to soft tissue windows. Scrolling down from top to bottom, be sure to look for any soft tissue swelling, lymph node enlargement, cardiac vasculature taking special note of the great vessels. In terms of the great vessels, the aortic arch will come into view first. Following the aorta down, one will note that it originates from the left ventricle and the distal aorta will be present slightly ventral and to the left of the vertebra. Pulmonary artery will be immediately below the aortic arch. Further down, pulmonary veins will be present. The SVC and IVC will be present toward the right side of the chest cavity ventral and lateral to the trachea and esophagus for the SVC and IVC, respectively.

On bone windows, be sure to check for rib fractures by scrolling up and down for each rib. Fractures will be noted by disruptions in the cortical surfaces. The vertebral bodies should also be noted for any fractures or disc herniations.

CT: Abdomen/Pelvis

CT of the abdomen and pelvis are usually obtained together to check for abdominal or pelvic pathology. Unlike the chest where the diaphragm serves to provide a separation of chest cavity organs from abdominal organ, no such barrier exists in the lower abdomen to separate lower abdominal organs from pelvic organs. Therefore, it is best to obtain these two body cavities together.

One approach in interpreting a CT abdomen/pelvis is to check each organ in a cranial to caudal fashion. The liver is inspected for any inhomogeneity including any masses or cysts. The bile ducts are inspected for dilation or obstruction. Gallbladder, if present, is inspected for wall thickening or presence of gallstones. Spleen is checked for masses or cysts. The stomach is inspected for signs of wall thickening or perforation/ulceration. Pancreas is analyzed for any masses or cysts. The pancreatic duct is checked for dilation and for any obstructing mass if dilated. The mesenteric vessels can be checked for any obvious abnormalities, however, only a dedicated CTA will be able to assess the mesenteric vessels to their full extent.

Following the small bowel will take some practice. One needs to follow the lumen of the small bowel while moving up and down as needed on the axial view. Transition points in small bowel obstruction can be identified by noticing a sudden decrease in the diameter of the bowel. Large bowel is easier to follow as it travels a more linear path along the lateral retroperitoneal areas and across the upper aspect of the peritoneum as the transverse segment. Diverticula will be noted as small outpouchings in the large bowel especially in the sigmoid colon region.

Kidneys and adrenal glands should be assessed for cysts or masses. Renal stones will appear as an opaque lesion within the renal pelvis or anywhere along the urinary tract. Bladder should be checked for any wall thickening or masses. In females, ovaries and uterus will be posterior to the bladder and should be checked for any cysts or masses. In males, the prostate can be visualized for enlargement or other focal masses. The splenic, para-aortic, mesenteric, iliac, inguinal, and femoral lymph nodes should be checked for enlargement.

The bony structures including the lower thoracic, lumbar spines, sacrum, coccyx, pelvis should be checked for any fractures or other abnormalities. The abdominal wall and soft tissues need to be carefully screened for hernias or fat stranding indicative of infection or inflammation.

Contrast Material

Contrast is used in plain film applications. Most common usage is in imaging of the GI tract. Barium or water-soluble material such as Gastrografin may be used in these imaging procedures.

Contrast is utilized frequently during CT and MR examinations to enhance visualization of organs such as the GI tract or blood vessels. In CT, iodine-based contrast is used when intravenous contrast is needed. Iodine contrast has evolved over the years, starting out with ionic high osmolar contrast to nonionic low osmolar contrast. Nonionic low osmolar contrast materials are safer to use with less adverse events. For oral contrast during CT examinations, barium is used most often.

Intravenous MR contrast is predominantly composed of gadolinium-chelated compounds. Copper and manganese have been used in the past; however, currently gadolinium is the most widely used. Nongadolinium base contrasts are used in selective MR imaging for various organs.

Adverse reactions to contrast materials include pruritus, hypotension, bronchospasm, to even life-threatening convulsions and pulmonary edema. Clinicians should monitor patients at greater risk for adverse reactions including those who have had reactions in the past, history of asthma or bronchospasm, history of allergy, or cardiac disease.

At our institution, a protocol exists for premedicating patient identified to be at high risk for adverse reactions. For planned contrast administration, give prednisone for 24 hours prior to CT scan (prednisone 50 mg q6h ×4 doses with the last dose given one hour before the scheduled scan time). For acute, emergent contrast administration, hydrocortisone 200 mg IV 1 hour prior and 3 hours post contrast injection and diphenhydramine 50 mg IV 1 hour prior to contrast administration is recommended. For pediatric contrast administration, prednisone 0.5 to 0.7 mg/kg PO (up to 50 mg) 7 hours, 3 hours, and 1 hour prior to contrast administration and diphenhydramine 1.25 mg/kg PO (up to 50 mg) 1 hour prior to contrast administration is recommended.

Protocols also exist for patient who experience adverse reactions after contrast administration. For mild reactions, IV hydration with normal saline or lactated Ringer 1 to 2 L, as well as diphenhydramine and hydrocortisone are recommended. For severe reactions, administration of epinephrine is recommended.

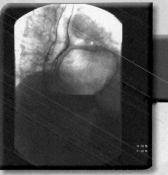

Esophagus

Esophageal Carcinoma

Overview

- Adenocarcinoma
  - Most common esophageal cancer in the United States
  - More common in the lower third of the esophagus
- Squamous cell carcinoma
  - Most common esophageal cancer worldwide
  - More common in the upper third of the esophagus

Risk Factors

- Tobacco use
- Heavy alcohol use
- Barrett esophagus
- Caustic injury

Signs and Symptoms

- Dysphagia and odynophagia
- Weight loss
- Midsternal chest pain
- Hoarseness of voice
- Early esophageal cancer is usually asymptomatic

Diagnosis

- Esophagogram
- Endoscopy with biopsy

- Endoscopic ultrasound for staging purposes-assess the depth of invasion and involvement of regional nodes
- Bronchoscopy to assess for airway invasion
- CT of the chest, abdomen, and pelvis for staging purposes
- PET scan to evaluate local and distant metastasis

Treatment

- Depending on the stage of the disease, treatment may include surgery, chemotherapy, and radiation therapy
- Advanced disease with dysphagia—may palliate symptoms with esophageal stent placement, laser therapy, or electrocoagulation

---

KEY POINT

- Remember that the esophagus has no serosal layer, so invasion to adjacent structures (trachea, aorta, pericardium) is common

---

RADIOLOGY

- **Plain film findings**
  - Air-fluid level within the superior mediastinum with widening of the azygoesophageal line
- **Esophagram findings**
  - Focal strictures with irregular borders/abrupt shoulder margins
  - Can also appear as long tubular filling defects similar to esophageal varices, but do not change with patient positioning
  - There may be stiffening of the mucosa and failure to collapse completely after the peristaltic wave passes, unlike achalasia
  - In contrast, leiomyomas and gastrointestinal stromal tumors (GISTs) are smooth wide-based, submucosal filling defects that form obtuse angles with the normal esophagus

- **CT findings** (Fig. 1.1)
  - Mainly used in the staging of esophageal cancer
    - Mediastinal lymphadenopathy
    - Effacement of the surrounding mediastinal fat, representing local invasion
  - Although nonspecific, there may be thickening of the esophageal wall
  - Dilated esophagus cranial to the lesion due to obstruction
- **PET/CT findings**
  - Hypermetabolic soft tissue within the esophagus
  - More sensitive and specific than CT in identifying lymphadenopathy and overall staging
- **Endoscopic US findings**
  - Carcinoma appears as a hypoechoic mass which interrupts the layers of the esophageal wall

FIGURE 1.1 A,B

A. Vertebra

B. Descending aorta

C. Heart

D. Stomach

E. Small bowel loops

F. Psoas muscle

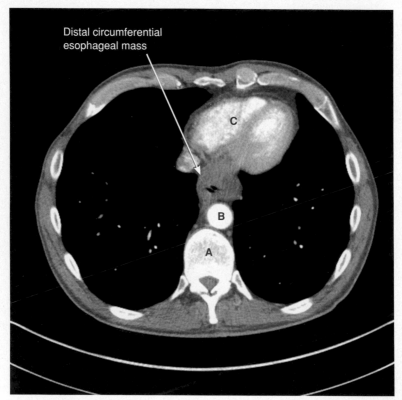

FIGURE 1.1 A

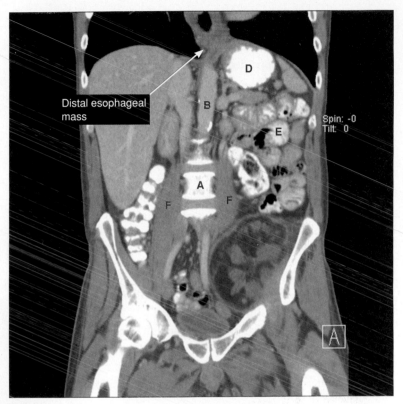

Distal esophageal mass

D

B

E

Spin: -0
Tilt: 0

A

F   F

A

FIGURE 1.1 B

Hiatal Hernia

Overview

Part of the stomach protrudes through a gap in the diaphgram, ending in the chest

Signs and Symptoms

- Mostly asymptomatic
- Gastroesophageal reflux symptoms: Heartburn, chest pain, sore throat, hoarseness of voice, bitter taste at the back of the mouth
- Other symptoms: Shortness of breath, dysphagia, epigastric discomfort, adult onset asthma, aspiration pneumonia, anemia (Cameron ulcers)

Classification of Hiatal Hernia (Fig. 1.2)

- Type I—most common; sliding hernia, herniation of the gastric cardia, displaced GE junction
- Type II—paraesophageal hernia, herniation of gastric fundus and body, GE junction normal in location
- Type III—combination of type I and II
- Type IV—herniation of the stomach and other abdominal organs, displaced GE junction

Diagnosis

- Upper GI series with barium contrast
- Upper endoscopy
- 24-hour esophageal pH testing
- Esophageal manometry

Treatment

- PPI and H2 blockers may help with symptomatic relief of heartburn
- Surgery is offered to patients who are symptomatic despite medical management

- Type I: Nissen fundoplication
- Type II–IV: Reduction of the herniated contents and Nissen/Toupet fundoplication

FIGURE 1.2

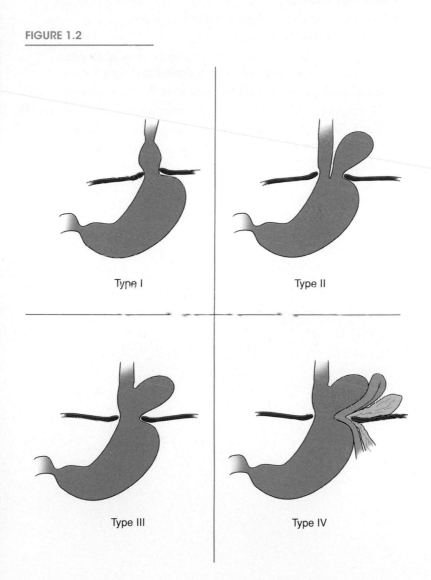

Type I

Type II

Type III

Type IV

RADIOLOGY

Sliding Hiatal Hernia

- **Plain film findings**
  - Large air collection overlying the heart shadow
- **Upper GI series findings** (Fig. 1.3)
  - A portion of the opacified stomach may be seen in the chest, changing in size and configuration during the examination
  - Gastroesophageal junction located above the diaphragm
  - GE junction is identified by the converging proximal gastric folds
  - May be associated with gastroesophageal reflux which may be witnessed during the examination
- **CT findings**
  - Displacement of a part of the stomach into the chest through the esophageal hiatus

FIGURE 1.3 A,B

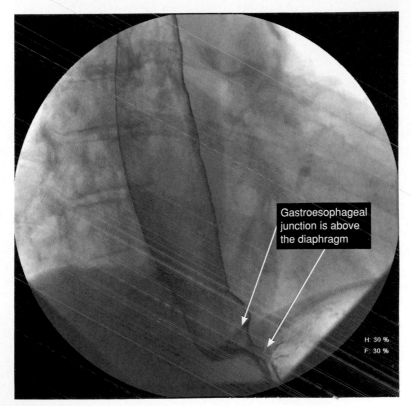

FIGURE 1.3 A

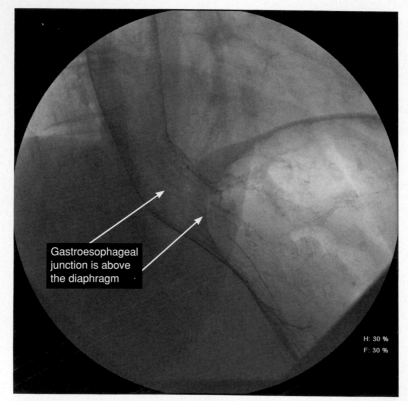

Gastroesophageal
junction is above
the diaphragm

H: 30 %
F: 30 %

FIGURE 1.3 B

Paraesophageal Hernia

- **Upper GI series findings** (Fig. 1.4)
  - Proximal stomach herniated lateral to the normal esophageal hiatus
  - More prone to incarceration and obstruction than a sliding hiatal hernia
- **CT findings** (Fig. 1.4)
  - Gastroesophageal junction located below the diaphragm
  - Proximal portion of stomach herniated usually to the left of the distal esophagus

FIGURE 1.4 A–D

A. Vertebra
B. Liver
C. Heart
D. Descending aorta
E. Aortic arch

F. Pulmonary artery
G. Left atrium
H. Bronchus
I. Spleen

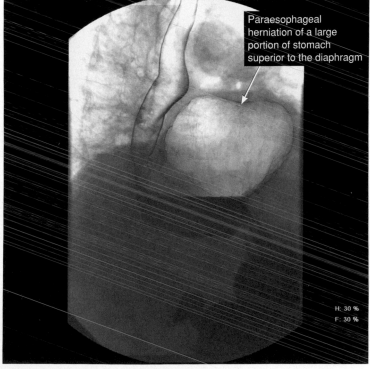

Paraesophageal herniation of a large portion of stomach superior to the diaphragm

H: 30 %
F: 30 %

FIGURE 1.4 A

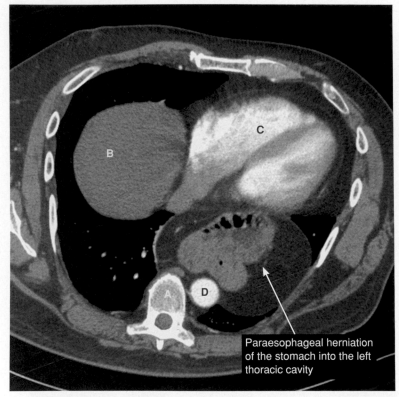

Paraesophageal herniation of the stomach into the left thoracic cavity

FIGURE 1.4 B

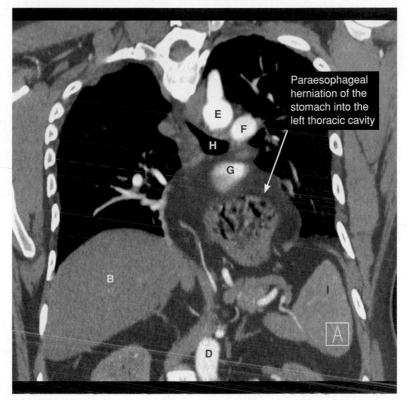

Paraesophageal herniation of the stomach into the left thoracic cavity

FIGURE 1.4 C

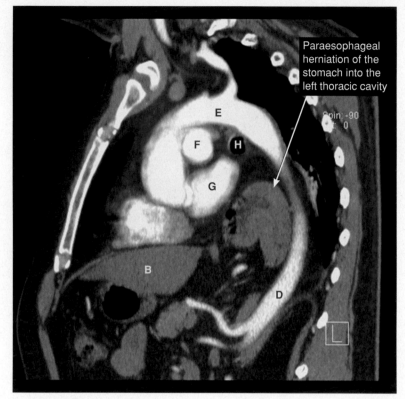

Paraesophageal herniation of the stomach into the left thoracic cavity

FIGURE 1.4 D

Status Post Nissen Fundoplication

- **Upper GI findings** (Fig. 1.5)
  - Subdiaphragmatic circumferential narrowing of the distal esophagus and gastroesophageal junction adjacent to surgical clips if placed from the surgery
- **CT findings**
  - Stomach wrapped 360 degrees around distal esophagus and gastroesophageal junction

FIGURE 1.5

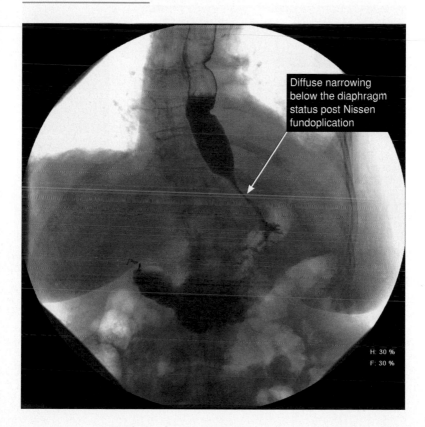

Diffuse narrowing below the diaphragm status post Nissen fundoplication

H: 30 %
F: 30 %

Slipped Nissen

- **Upper GI findings** (Fig. 1.6)
  - Type I consists of paraesophageal herniation of a portion of Nissen wrap through the esophageal hiatus
  - Type II consists of herniation of entire Nissen wrap through the esophageal hiatus

FIGURE 1.6 A,B

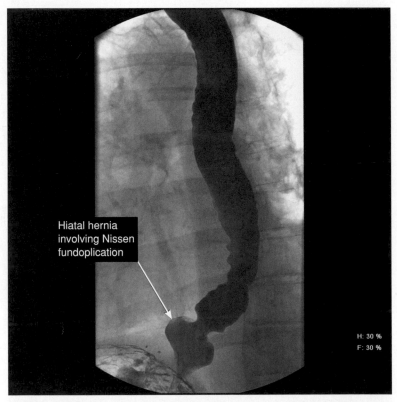

Hiatal hernia involving Nissen fundoplication

H: 30 %
F: 30 %

FIGURE 1.6 A

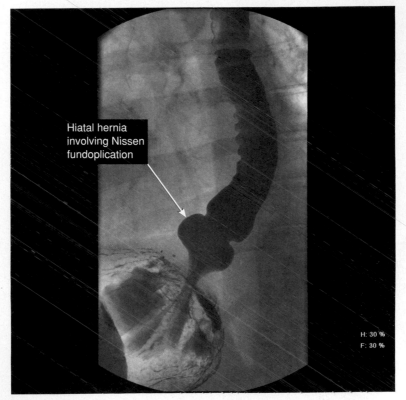

Hiatal hernia involving Nissen fundoplication

H: 30 %
F: 30 %

FIGURE 1.6 B

Suggested Readings

Abbara S, Kalan MM, Lewicki AM. Intrathoracic stomach revisited. *AJR Am J Roentgenol.* 2003;181:403–414.

Baker ME, Einstein DM, Herts BR, et al. Gastroesophageal reflux disease: Integrating the barium esophagram before and after antireflux surgery. *Radiology.* 2007; 243:329–339.

Canon CL, Morgan DE, Einstein DM, et al. Surgical approach to gastroesophageal reflux disease: What the radiologist needs to know. *Radiographics.* 2005;25:1485–1499.

Hainaux B, Sattari A, Coppens E, et al. Intrathoracic migration of the wrap after laparoscopic Nissen fundoplication: Radiologic evaluation. *AJR Am J Roentge* 2002;178:859–862.

Kim TJ, Kim HY, Lee KW, et al. Multimodality assessment of esophage cer: Preoperative staging and monitoring of response to therapy. *Radi* 2009;29:403–421.

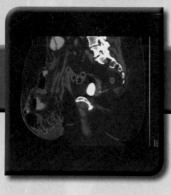

Hernias

Hernias occur when there is an anatomical defect or an area that is weakened, allowing abdominal contents such as small bowel, omentum, etc. to herniate.

KEY POINTS

- The most significant consequence of a hernia is incarceration of the herniated viscera that may lead to strangulation
- Strangulation may lead to bowel necrosis and is therefore a surgical emergency
  - Skin changes (redness) overlying the area of incarceration, severe tenderness, leukocytosis, and signs of sepsis are classical signs for strangulation
- Hernias with a small neck have increased risk of incarceration and strangulation compared to larger neck hernias

---

Incisional/Ventral Hernias

- Risk factors include previous abdominal surgeries, obesity, smoking, steroid usage
- Diagnosed when the hernia occurs in the vicinity of a prior incision

RADIOLOGY

Abdominal Incisional Hernia

- **CT findings** (Fig. 2.1)
  - Can occur within any part of the abdominal wall
  - Displacement of abdominal contents through the abdominal wall defect

FIGURE 2.1 A–C

A. Small bowel loops
B. Psoas muscle
C. Vertebra
D. Liver
E. Descending aorta

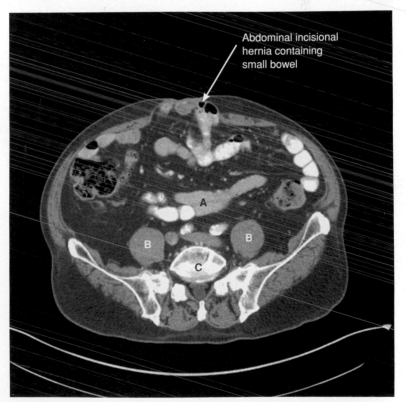

Abdominal incisional hernia containing small bowel

FIGURE 2.1 A

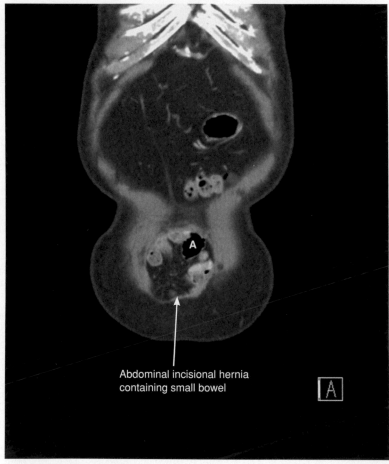

Abdominal incisional hernia
containing small bowel

FIGURE 2.1 B

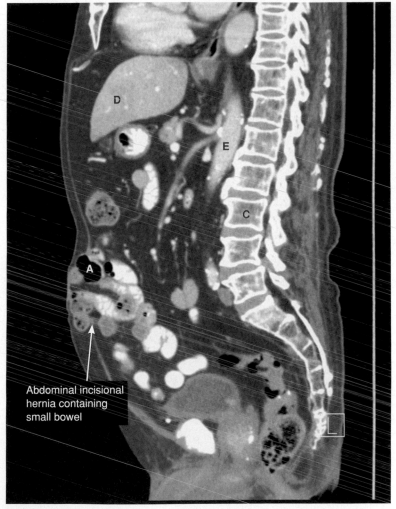

Abdominal incisional hernia containing small bowel

FIGURE 2.1 C

Incisional Hernia with Acutely Incarcerated Bowel—Dilated and Thickened

- **CT findings** (Fig. 2.2)
  - Thickened, edematous bowel loops with or without dilated proximal loops indicating obstruction
  - Fat stranding may be noted in the mesentery within the incisional hernia, indicating venous congestion or inflammation
  - Incarceration is suggested when herniation is associated with thickened bowel loops within the hernia with or without dilated bowel loops located proximal to the hernia

FIGURE 2.2 A–C

A. Rectum   C. Small bowel loops
B. Bladder   D. Vertebra

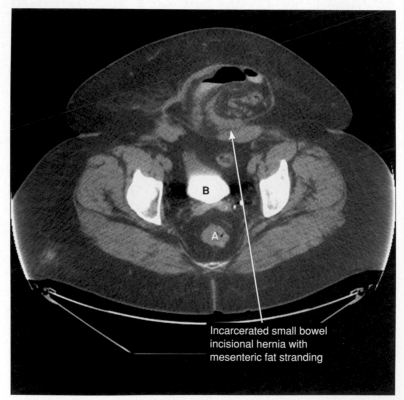

Incarcerated small bowel incisional hernia with mesenteric fat stranding

FIGURE 2.2 A

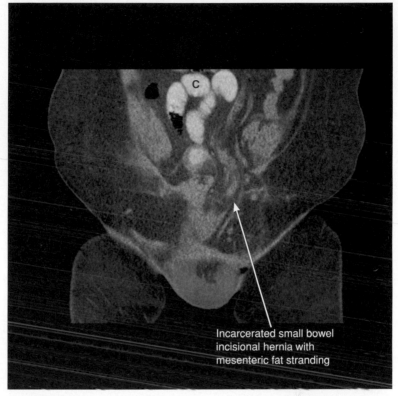

Incarcerated small bowel incisional hernia with mesenteric fat stranding

FIGURE 2.2 B

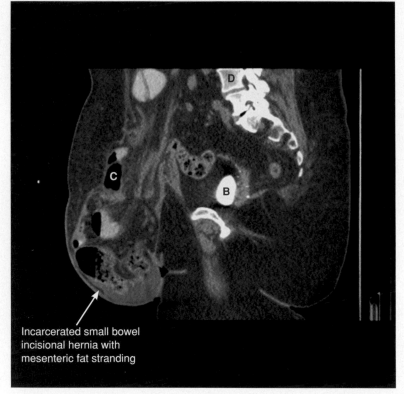

Incarcerated small bowel
incisional hernia with
mesenteric fat stranding

FIGURE 2.2 C

Status Post Ventral Hernia Repair

- **CT findings** (Fig. 2.3)
  - Depending on how the repair was performed, the postoperative abdomen will contain either:
    - Staples which are small hyperdensities with streak artifact
    - Polypropylene (PP) mesh which are not usually visualized because its density is similar to soft tissue
    - Polytetrafluoroethylene (PTFE) mesh which appear as linear areas of high density

FIGURE 2.3 A–C

A. Liver   D. Vertebra
B. Gallbladder E. Small bowel loops
C. Kidney

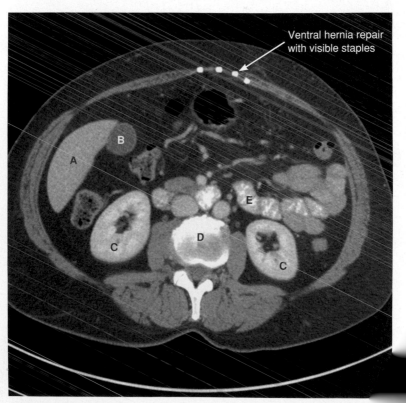

Ventral hernia repair with visible staples

FIGURE 2.3 A

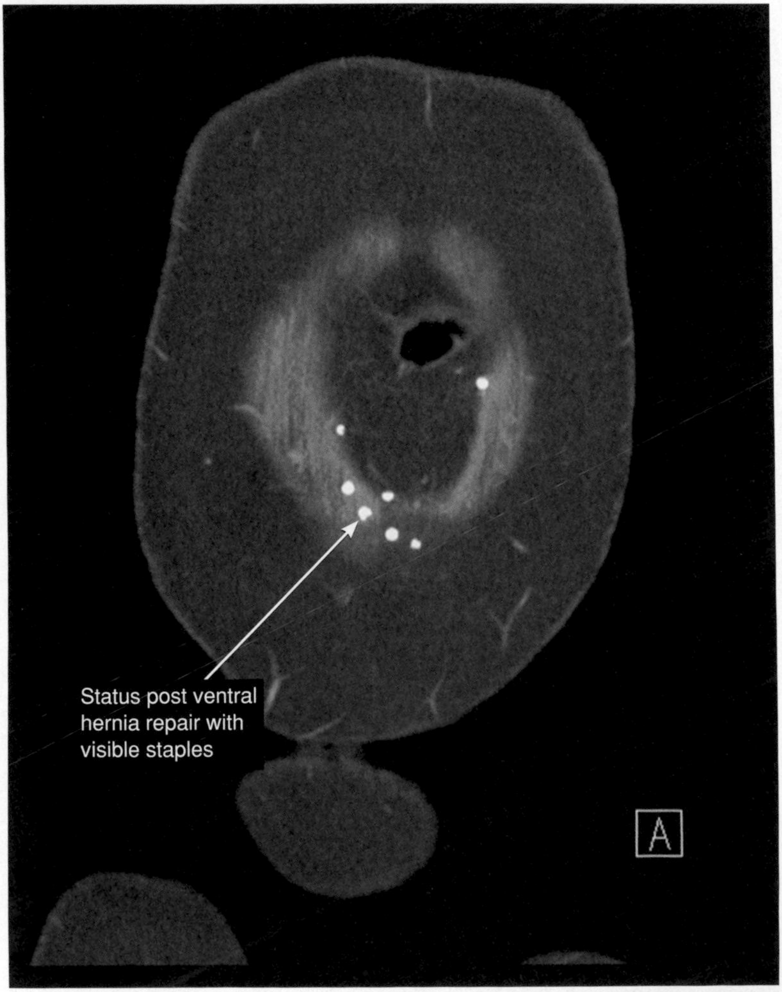

Status post ventral
hernia repair with
visible staples

FIGURE 2.3 B

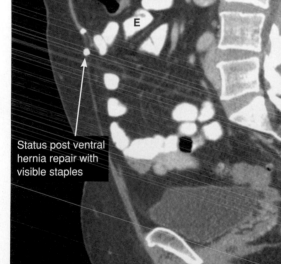

Status post ventral hernia repair with visible staples

FIGURE 2.3 C

Status Post Ventral Hernia Repair—Infected Mesh with Abscess

- **CT findings** (Fig. 2.4)
  - Fluid or phlegmon adjacent to the site of the hernia repair
  - Because superficial fluid collections are usually treated conservatively, superficial collections must be differentiated from deep collections
  - Gas or septa may develop in a fluid collection
  - Aspiration of fluid collection is often need to make the diagnosis

FIGURE 2.4 A,B

A. Small bowel loops

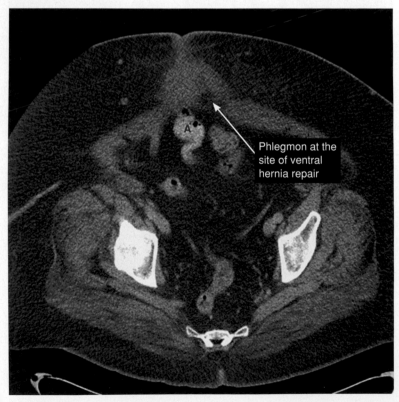

Phlegmon at the site of ventral hernia repair

FIGURE 2.4 A

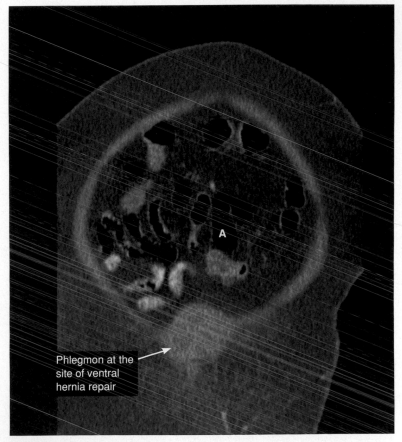

FIGURE 2.4 B

Flank Incisional Hernia

■ **CT findings** (Fig. 2.5)

- Protrusion of mesentery, bowel loops, or other abdominal organs through the lateral abdominal wall defect

FIGURE 2.5 A,B

A. Kidney   D. Liver
B. Small bowel   E. Iliopsoas muscle
C. Vertebra

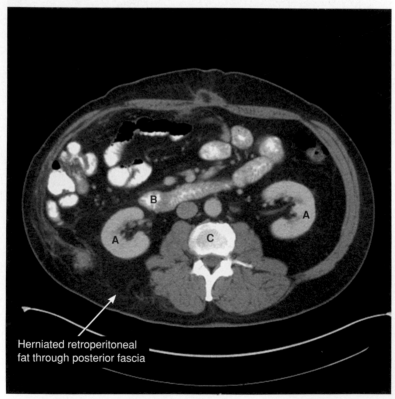

Herniated retroperitoneal
fat through posterior fascia

FIGURE 2.5 A

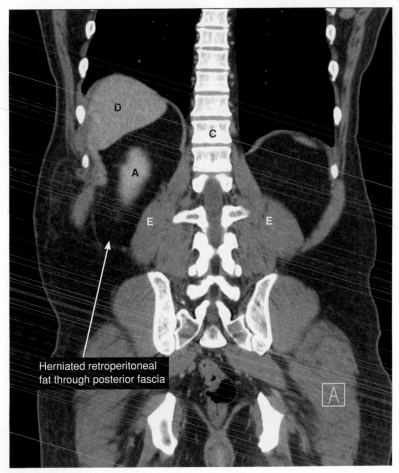

FIGURE 2.5 B

Diaphragmatic Hernia

- Usually left-sided, with the stomach and bowels protruding through the diaphragmatic defect and into the chest
- Can be congenital (Bochdalek = posterolateral, Morgagni = anteromedial), or traumatic in etiology

RADIOLOGY

Diaphragmatic Hernia—Morgagni Hernia

- **Plain film findings** (Fig. 2.6)
  - Anterior opacity at cardiophrenic angle best seen on the frontal view
  - Difficult to differentiate from an anterior mediastinal mass such as a pericardial cyst
- **CT findings**
  - Herniation of the abdominal contents through an anterior defect in the diaphragm
  - Can contain omentum, bowel loops, or liver

FIGURE 2.6 A–E

A. Heart
B. Descending aorta
C. Vertebra
D. Liver
E. Gallbladder
F. Small bowel loops
G. Stomach
H. Psoas muscle

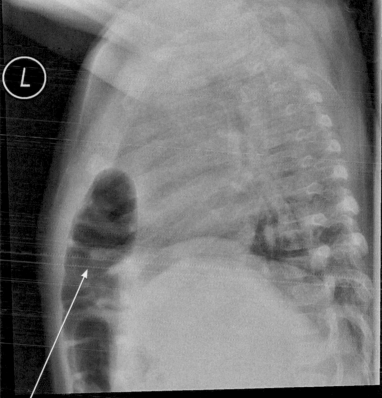

Congenital diaphragmatic hernia

CROSS-TABLE

LATERAL

FIGURE 2.6 A

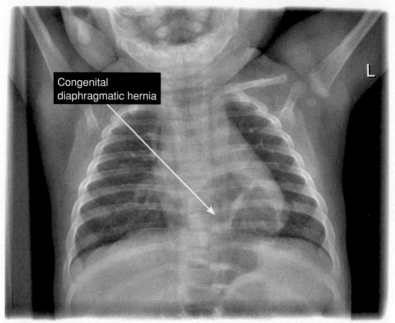

Congenital diaphragmatic hernia

L

FIGURE 2.6 B

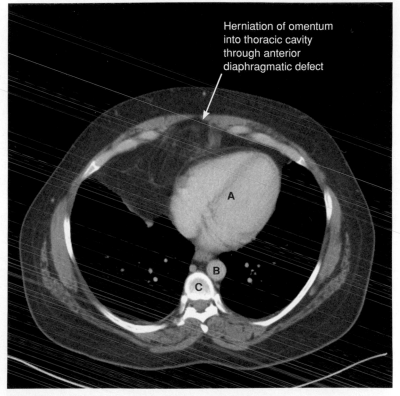

FIGURE 2.6 C

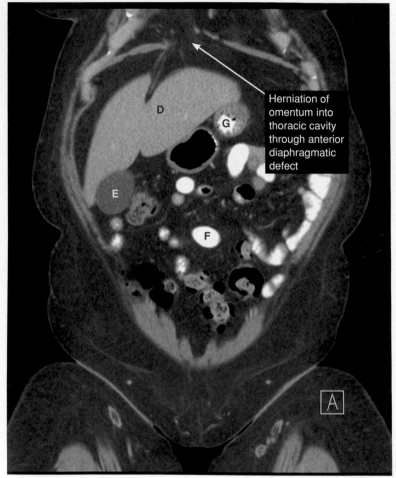

Herniation of omentum into thoracic cavity through anterior diaphragmatic defect

FIGURE 2.6 D

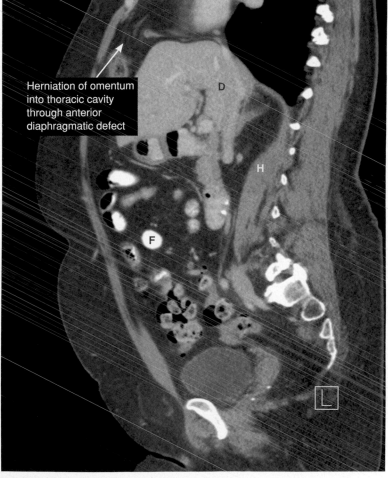

Herniation of omentum into thoracic cavity through anterior diaphragmatic defect

FIGURE 2.6 E

Diaphragmatic Hernia—Bochdalek Hernia

- **Plain film findings**
  - Soft tissue opacity with or without bowel gas overlying the lower hemithorax
- **CT findings** (Fig. 2.7)
  - Herniation of abdominal contents through a defect usually in the posterior aspect of the diaphragm
  - May contain portions of the stomach, retroperitoneal fat, spleen or kidney
  - Majority occurs on the left

FIGURE 2.7 A–C

A. Liver
B. Descending aorta
C. Vertebra

D. Psoas muscle
E. Kidney
F. Small bowel loops

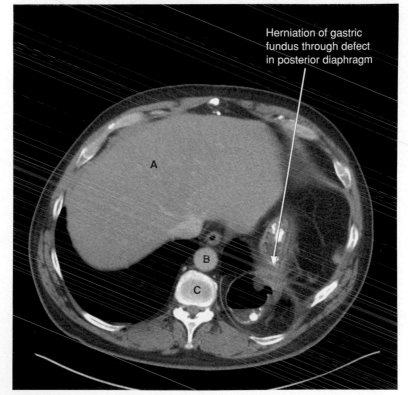

Herniation of gastric fundus through defect in posterior diaphragm

FIGURE 2.7 A

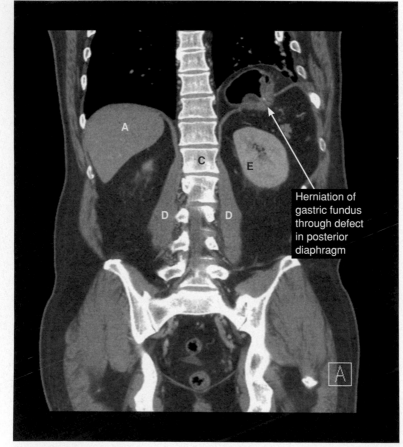

Herniation of gastric fundus through defect in posterior diaphragm

FIGURE 2.7 B

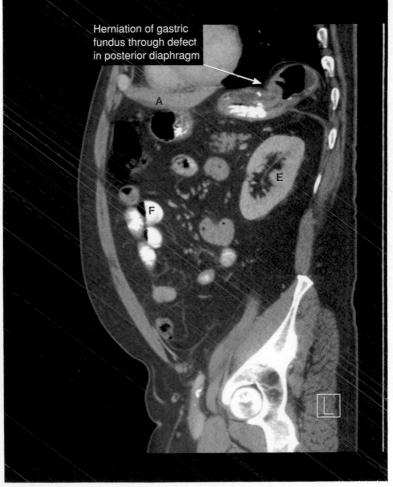

Herniation of gastric fundus through defect in posterior diaphragm

A

E

F

L

FIGURE 2.7 C

Inguinal Hernia

■ Understand the basic anatomy of the inguinal region and Hesselbach's triangle
  • Rectus sheath, inferior epigastric artery, and the inguinal ligament
■ **Direct**—through the Hesselbach's triangle, medial to the inferior epigastric vessels
  Indirect—lateral to the inferior epigastric vessels
■ Usually presents as a bulge in the groin and may enlarge upon Valsalva maneuver (cough, defecation, heavy lifting)

RADIOLOGY

Bilateral Inguinal Hernia

■ **CT findings** (Fig. 2.8)
  • Direct inguinal hernia is diagnosed by bowel loops, or omentum protruding through the inguinal canal medial to the inferior epigastric vessels
  • Indirect inguinal hernia is diagnosed by bowel loops, omentum, or omental fat protruding through the inguinal canal lateral to the inferior epigastric vessels, and potentially into the scrotum

FIGURE 2.8 A–D

A. Bladder   E. Gallbladder
B. Rectum   F. Stomach
C. Femoral head   G. Small bowel loops
D. Liver   H. Vertebra

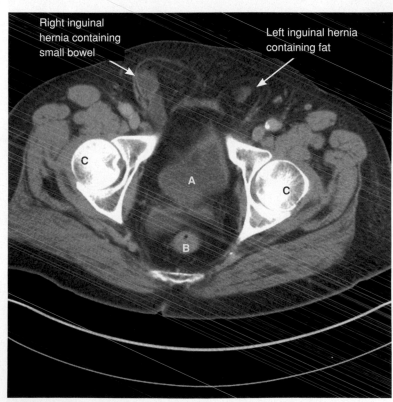

FIGURE 2.8 A

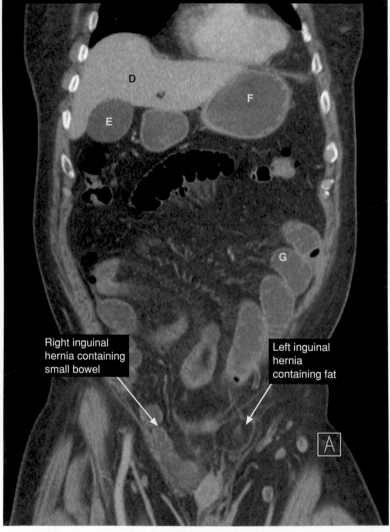

FIGURE 2.8 B

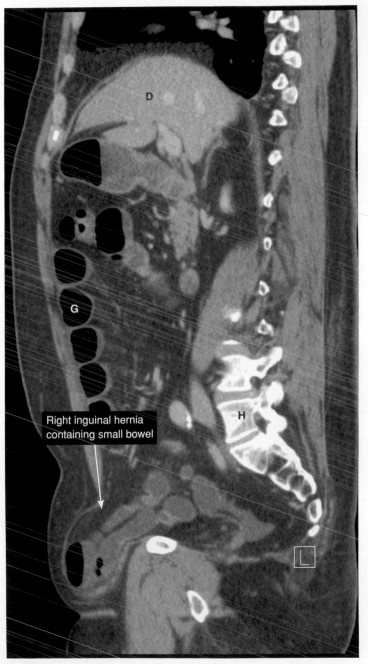

Right inguinal hernia
containing small bowel

FIGURE 2.8 C

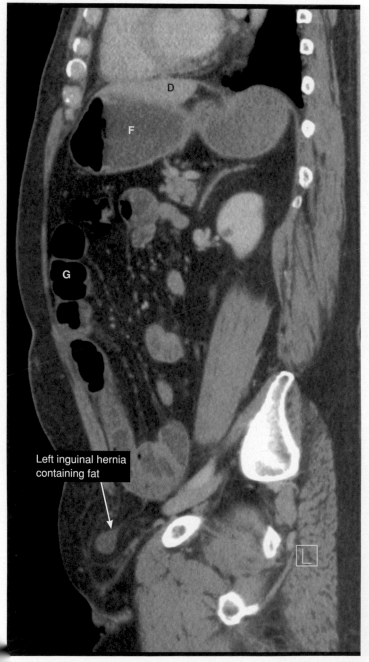

Left inguinal hernia containing fat

FIGURE 2.8 D

Incarcerated Inguinal Hernia

- **CT findings** (Fig. 2.9)
  - Omental fat or bowel loops passing through the inguinal canal and into the scrotum
  - Edema and inflammation within the hernia sac can be seen

FIGURE 2.9 A–C

A. Bladder

B. Rectum

C. Femoral head

D. Liver

E. Small bowel loops

F. Stomach

G. Gallbladder

H. Kidney

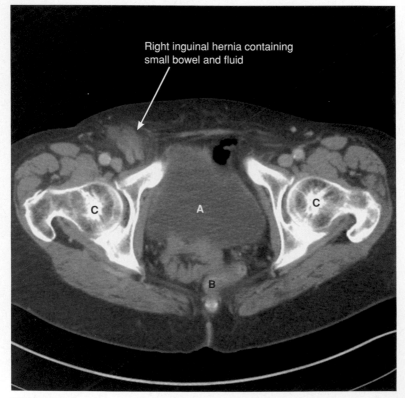

Right inguinal hernia containing small bowel and fluid

FIGURE 2.9 A

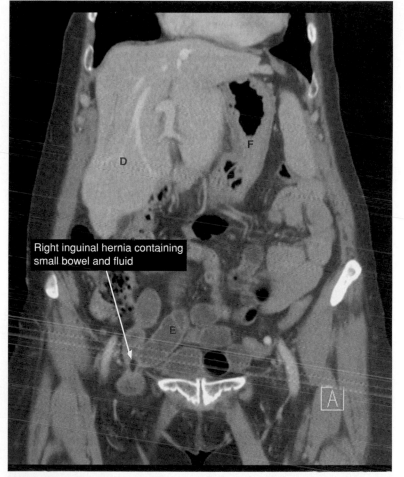

FIGURE 2.9 B

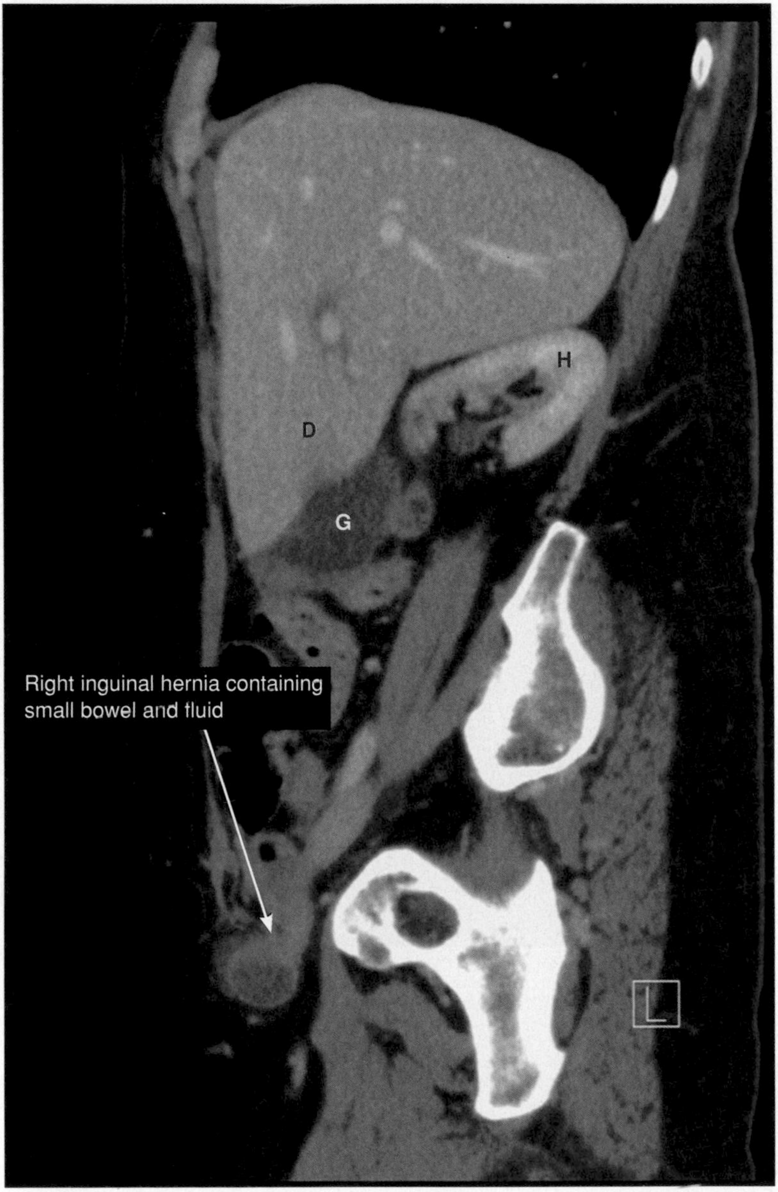

Right inguinal hernia containing small bowel and fluid

FIGURE 2.9 C

Parastomal Hernia

- Formation of a stoma requires the creation of a defect in the abdominal wall
- Parastomal hernia is a result of progressive enlargement of the defect, leading to herniation of bowel contents adjacent to the ostomy site

RADIOLOGY

- **CT findings** (Fig. 2.10)
  - Similar to an incisional hernia
  - Omentum or bowel protruding next to the ostomy site
  - Usually difficult to detect on physical examination

FIGURE 2.10 A–C

A. Small bowel loops   D. Liver
B. Psoas muscle   E. Stomach
C. Vertebra   F. Kidney

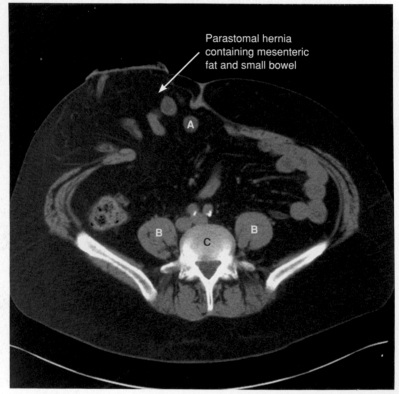

Parastomal hernia containing mesenteric fat and small bowel

FIGURE 2.10 A

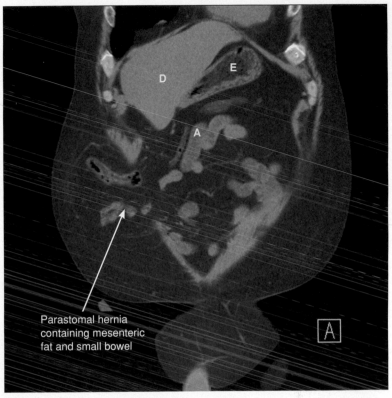

Parastomal hernia
containing mesenteric
fat and small bowel

FIGURE 2.10 B

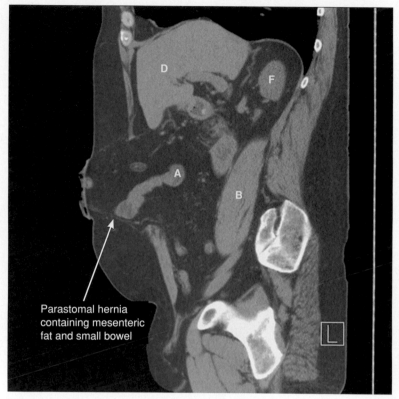

Parastomal hernia containing mesenteric fat and small bowel

FIGURE 2.10 C

Umbilical Hernia

- A common hernia seen in the pediatric population
  - Many will resolve by the age of 3 or 4 years
  - Consider surgery if the hernia does not resolve by the age of 4 years, if the size is big/enlarging, or if there is concern for bowel incarceration.
- Also a common hernia seen in the adult due to obesity, pregnancy, ascites, smoking, chronic cough

RADIOLOGY

- **CT findings** (Fig. 2.11)
  - Omentum or bowel loops protruding through the umbilical canal which is bordered by umbilical fascia posteriorly, linea alba anteriorly, and medial edges of the rectus sheaths on each side

FIGURE 2.11 A–C

A. Psoas muscle
B. Vertebra
C. Small bowel loops

D. Transverse colon
E. Bladder
F. Descending aorta

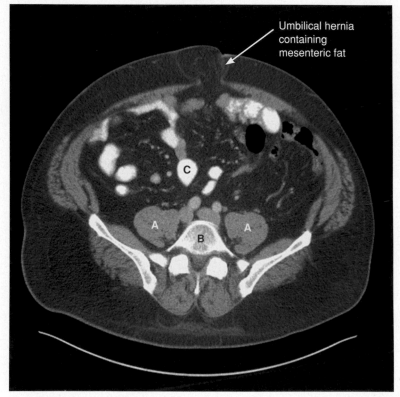

Umbilical hernia containing mesenteric fat

FIGURE 2.11 A

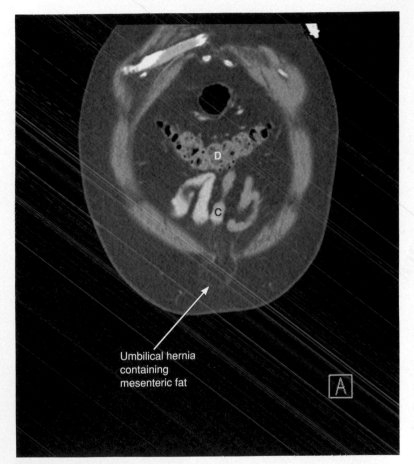

Umbilical hernia
containing
mesenteric fat

FIGURE 2.11 B

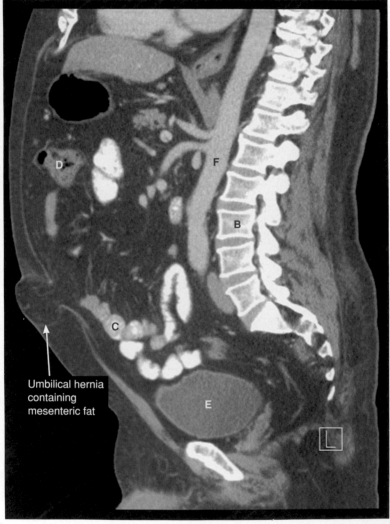

Umbilical hernia containing mesenteric fat

FIGURE 2.11 C

Suggested Readings

Aguirre DA, Casola G, Sirlin C. Abdominal wall hernias: MDCT findings. *AJR Am J Roentgenol.* 2004;183:681–690.

Aguirre DA, Santosa AC, Casola G, et al. Abdominal wall hernias: Imaging features, complications, and diagnostic pitfalls at multi-detector row CT. *Radiographics.* 2005;25:1501–1520.

Burkhardt JH, Arshanskiy Y, Munson JL, et al. Diagnosis of inguinal region hernias with axial CT: The lateral crescent sign and other key findings. *Radiographics.* 2011;31(2):E1–E12.

Gale ME. Bochdalek hernia: Prevalence and CT characteristics. *Radiology.* 1985; 156:449–452.

Mullins ME, Stein J, Saini SS, et al. Prevalence of incidental Bochdalek's hernia in a large adult population. *AJR Am J Roentgenol.* 2001;177:363–366.

Panicek DM, Benson CB, Gottlieb RH, et al. The diaphragm: Anatomic, pathologic, and radiologic considerations. *Radiographics.* 1988;8:385–425.

Parra JA, Revuelta S, Gallego T, et al. Prosthetic mesh used for inguinal and ventral hernia repair: Normal appearance and complications in ultrasound and CT. *Br J Radiol.* 2004;77:261–265.

Salameh JR. Primary and unusual abdominal wall hernias. *Surg Clin North Am.* 2008;88:45–60.

Shadbolt CL, Heinze SB, Dietrich RB. Imaging of groin masses: Inguinal anatomy and pathologic conditions revisited. *Radiographics.* 2001;21:S261–S271.

Zarvan NP, Lee FT Jr, Yandow DR, et al. Abdominal hernias: CT findings. *AJR Am J Roentgenol.* 1995;164:1391–1395.

Zausner J, Dumont AE, Ring SM. Obturator hernia. *Am J Roentgenol Radium Ther Nucl Med.* 1972;115(2):408–410.

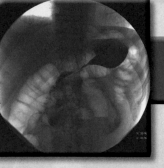

Stomach

Gastric Neoplasms

Overview

- Adenocarcinoma (>90%), gastric lymphoma (~3% to 5%), gastrointestinal stromal tumors (GISTs) (~3%)

Clinical Presentation

- Weight loss, early satiety, abdominal pain, nausea, vomiting
- Dysphagia if tumor is in the proximal stomach (cardia)
- Gastric adenocarcinoma metastasis
  - Virchow's node: Metastasis to the left supraclavicular node
  - Sister Mary Joseph nodule: Metastasis to the periumbilical region
  - Krukenberg tumor: Metastasis to the ovary
  - Blumer's shelf: Metastasis to the pouch of Douglas

Diagnosis

- EGD is the gold standard for tissue diagnosis
- EUS to assess for depth of invasion and lymphadenopathy
- CT abdomen/pelvis and CXR for staging purposes

Treatment

- **Adenocarcinoma**
  - Diagnostic laparoscopy to assess for metastatic disease
  - Surgical resection with 5 cm margins with D1 or D2 nodal dissection
  - Neoadjuvant or adjuvant chemotherapy depending on the stage
- **Lymphoma**
  - All are nonHodgkin type, most are low grade MALT (mucosal associated lymph tissue)
  - Low-grade MALT: Likely a result of chronic *Helicobacter pylori* infection
    - Antibiotic treatment for *H. pylori*
    - Radiation ± chemotherapy for persistent disease after *H. pylori* treatment
  - High-grade MALT: Chemotherapy and radiation therapy
- **GIST**
  - Arises from interstitial cells of Cajal (intestinal pacemaker cells)
  - Due to *c-kit* mutation
  - Resection with negative margins
  - Consider imatinib (Gleevec) if
    - tumor >5 cm in size
    - more than 5 mitotic figures per 50 high-power field
    - nongastric location
    - tumor rupture
    - KIT—positive unresectable, metastatic, or recurrent disease

RADIOLOGY

Gastric Cancer

- **Plain film findings**
  - Gastric mass is usually not seen on plain radiographs
  - Omental calcified metastases may sometimes be visible

- **Upper GI findings**
  - If small, gastric adenocarcinomas will manifest as a raised ulcer with surrounding mucosal edema
    - Folds are often thickened, irregular, or nodular
    - Ulcerations, if present, are irregular in shape and do not extend beyond the gastric lumen
    - If the antrum is involved, it may be severely narrowed or obstructed
- **CT findings** (Fig. 3.1)
  - Focal wall thickening with or without ulceration, mass, or diffuse wall thickening
  - CT is superior to barium studies to evaluate for the extent of disease
  - Extension of tumor into adjacent organs and omental carcinomatosis can be seen
  - Presence or absence of regional lymphadenopathy (adenopathy in the left gastric, porta hepatis, and peripancreatic regions) and presence of liver metastases can be evaluated

FIGURE 3.1

A. Liver

B. Descending aorta

C. Vertebra

D. Spleen

E. Splenic cyst

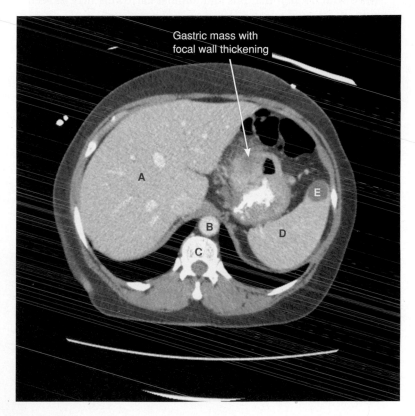

Gastric mass with focal wall thickening

Gastric Lymphoma

- **Upper GI findings**
  - Focal or diffuse gastric fold thickening
  - Mass with nodular margins and luminal narrowing may be seen
- **CT findings** (Fig. 3.2)
  - Focal or diffuse fold thickening, which can be associated with regional lymphadenopathy

FIGURE 3.2 A–C

A. Liver
B. Kidney
C. IVC
D. Descending aorta

E. Vertebra
F. Spleen
G. Small bowel loops
H. Bladder

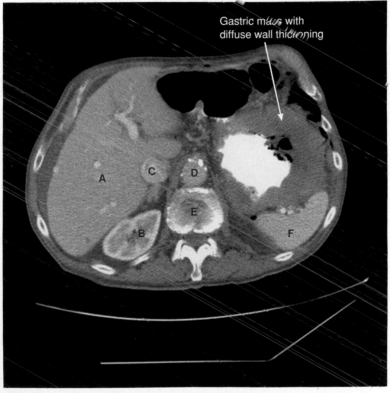

Gastric mass with
diffuse wall thickening

FIGURE 3.2 A

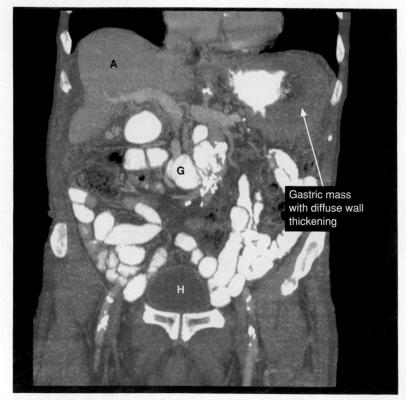

Gastric mass with diffuse wall thickening

FIGURE 3.2 B

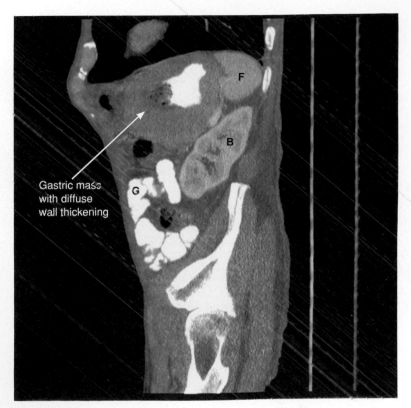

Gastric mass with diffuse wall thickening

FIGURE 3.2 C

GIST Tumor

- **Plain film findings**
  - Nonspecific mass indenting or displacing the gastric bubble may be seen
  - Upper GI Findings
    - ○ Intraluminal filling defect arising from the wall, forming smooth, obtuse angles with the rest of the stomach
- **CT findings** (Fig. 3.3)
  - Mass arising from the gastric wall, usually with an exophytic growth pattern
  - Central areas of low attenuation indicate hemorrhage or necrosis
- **MRI findings**
  - Solid portions of tumor are T1 hypointense (pre-contrast) and T2 hyperintense
  - Hemorrhage within tumor will manifest with variable T1 and T2 signals
  - Heterogeneous enhancement

FIGURE 3.3 A–C

A. Liver
B. Descending aorta
C. Vertebra
D. Spleen

E. IVC
F. Kidney
G. Psoas muscle
H. Adnexal cyst

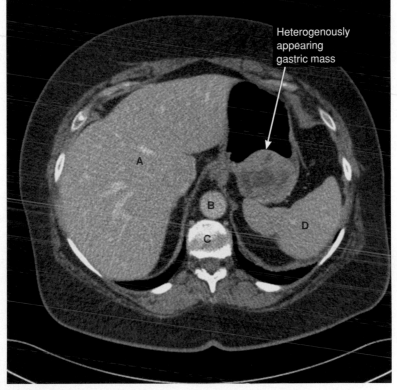

Heterogenously appearing gastric mass

FIGURE 3.3 A

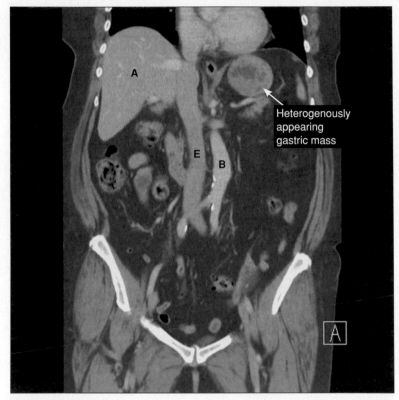

FIGURE 3.3 B

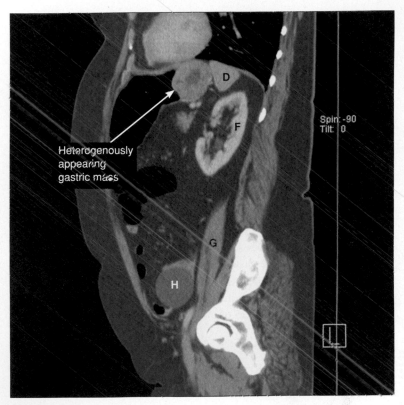

FIGURE 3.3 C

Gastric Outlet Obstruction

■ In adults, peptic ulcer disease (PUD) and gastric cancer account for more than 90% of gastric outlet obstruction with PUD being the most common cause

RADIOLOGY

■ **Plain film findings/upper GI findings** (Fig. 3.4)
  • Prominent gastric air bubble with a gastric air–fluid level and dilated stomach is seen
  • Narrowing of the gastric lumen
■ **CT findings** (Fig. 3.4)
  • Dilated stomach
  • Inflammatory diseases such as pancreatitis may cause inflammation of the gastric wall resulting in obstruction
  • Differentiation between benign and malignant cause of obstruction depends on the presence of inflammatory disease or a mass within the region of obstruction

FIGURE 3.4 A–C

A. Liver
B. Portal vein
C. IVC
D. Descending aorta

E. Vertebra
F. Spleen
G. Small bowel loops

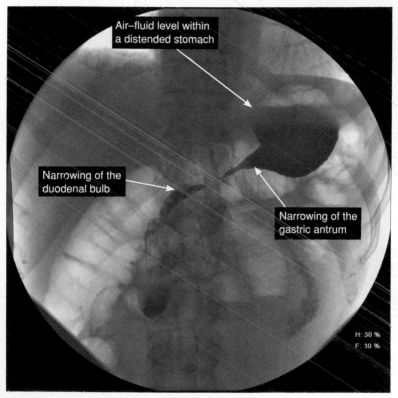

FIGURE 3.4 A

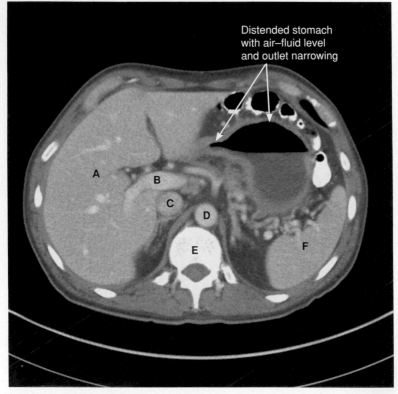

FIGURE 3.4 B

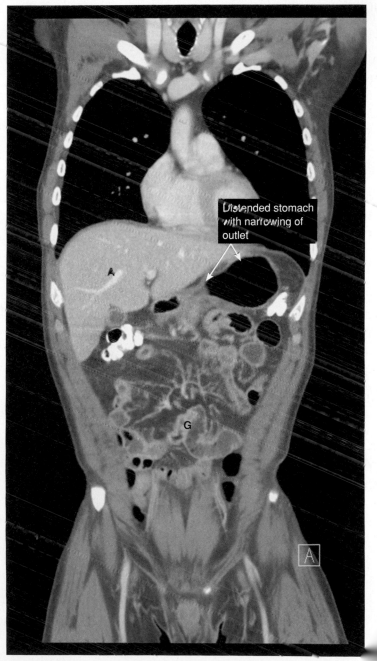

FIGURE 3.4 C

Pyloric Stenosis

Overview

- A congenital condition
- Hypertrophy of the muscles around the pylorus, causing gastric outlet obstruction
- Usually presents from 2 weeks to 3 months of age
- Most prevalent in first born males (males to females 4:1)

Clinical Presentation

- Nonbilious projectile emesis
- Hypochloremic, hypokalemic metabolic alkalosis with paradoxical aciduria
- Palpable "olive" in the epigastric region

Diagnosis

- Clinical diagnosis with confirmation made using ultrasound or an upper GI

Treatment

- Fluid resuscitation with normal saline to correct metabolic alkalosis
- Laparoscopic or open pyloromyotomy

RADIOLOGY

- **Upper GI findings**
  - Elongation of the pyloric channel (2 to 4 cm long) with smooth narrowing
  - Hypertrophied muscle may bulge retrograde into the gastric antrum creating a shoulder of contrast

- **US findings** (Fig. 3.5)
  - Channel length is longer than 15 mm
  - Transverse pyloric diameter is larger than 11 mm
  - Pyloric muscle wall thickness is greater than 2.5 mm
  - Small amounts of gastric emptying or large gastric residue is noted
- **CT findings**
  - Hypertrophy and hyperplasia of the circular muscle of the pylorus with some contribution of the longitudinal muscle
  - Hypertrophied muscle lengthens and narrows the pyloric channel

FIGURE 3.5 A,B

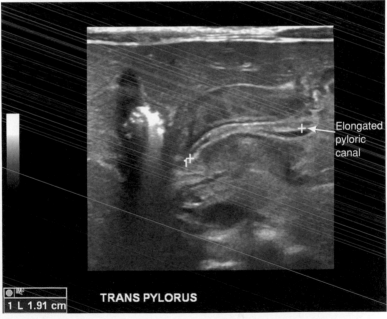

1 L 1.91 cm

TRANS PYLORUS

Elongated pyloric canal

FIGURE 3.5 A

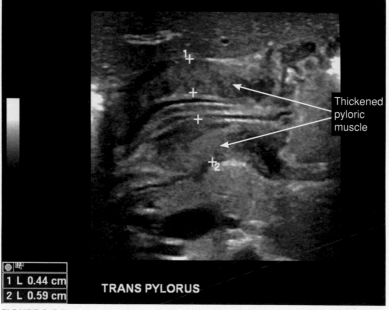

Thickened pyloric muscle

1 L 0.44 cm
2 L 0.59 cm

TRANS PYLORUS

FIGURE 3.5 B

Duodenal Ulcer/Gastric Perforation

Overview

- 70% to 90% are associated with *H. pylori* infection
- Other etiologies include NSAID use, Zollinger–Ellison syndrome, smoking, trauma, burn injury (Curling's ulcer)

Modified Johnson Classification of Peptic Ulcers

- Type I: Ulcer along the body of the stomach (mostly along lesser curvature)—Low to normal amount of acid
- Type II: Ulcer in the body of the stomach and duodenum—High acid
- Type III: Ulcer in the pyloric channel within 3 cm of the pylorus—High acid
- Type IV: Ulcer near the GE junction—Low to normal amount of acid
- Type V: Ulcer associated with NSAID use, may occur throughout the stomach

Signs and Symptoms

- Sudden onset of severe upper abdominal pain which may progress to diffuse peritonitis
- History of ulcer disease, previously treated for *H. pylori* infection, NSAID usage

Diagnosis

- Free air on abdominal x-ray
- Free air on abdominal pelvic CT scan with or without extravasation of oral contrast

Treatment/Management

- If only few dots of free air without contrast extravasation, may manage conservatively with serial abdominal examination, IV antibiotics, NPO
- Patients with diffuse peritonitis or sepsis will warrant operative exploration
- Workup for *H. pylori* infection

RADIOLOGY

- **Plain film findings** (Fig. 3.6)
  - Area of lucency below the right hemidiaphragm on upright abdominal films
  - Lucency lateral to the liver on left lateral decubitus views
  - Rigler's sign, which is defined as identifying both outer and inner walls of a bowel loop, may be seen with diffuse free air within the peritoneum on the supine view
    - Falciform or umbilical ligaments may be seen with diffuse free air
- **Upper GI findings**
  - Leak of water-soluble contrast within the peritoneal cavity
  - Site of perforation will vary depending on etiology
- **CT findings** (Fig. 3.6)
  - CT may be used to delineate questionable free air found on plain films
  - Discontinuity of wall on contrast-enhanced CT
  - Focal thickening of stomach wall next to extraluminal gas bubbles secondary to inflammation

FIGURE 3.6 A–F

A. Liver
B. IVC
C. Descending aorta
D. Vertebra
E. Contrast within lesser sac
F. Spleen
G. Kidney
H. Psoas muscle
I. Stomach

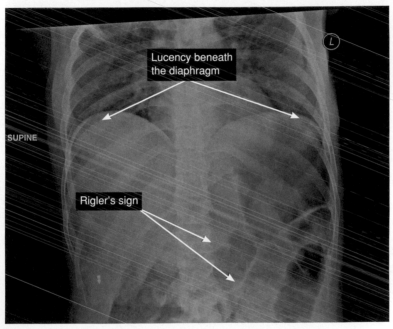

FIGURE 3.6 A

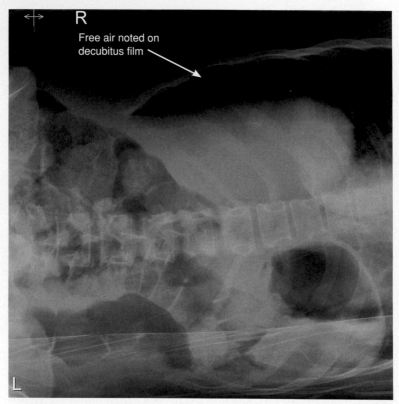

FIGURE 3.6 B

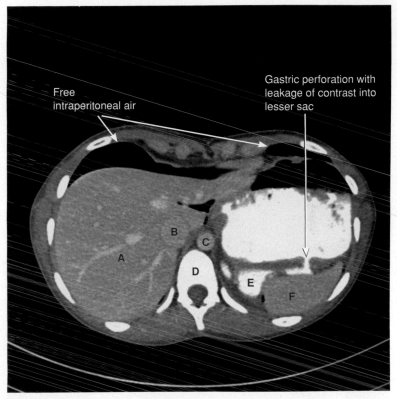

Free intraperitoneal air

Gastric perforation with leakage of contrast into lesser sac

FIGURE 3.6 C

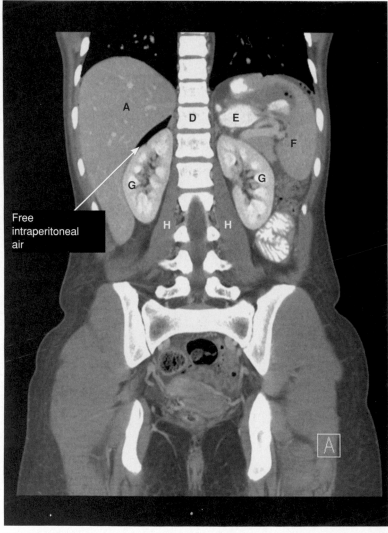

FIGURE 3.6 D

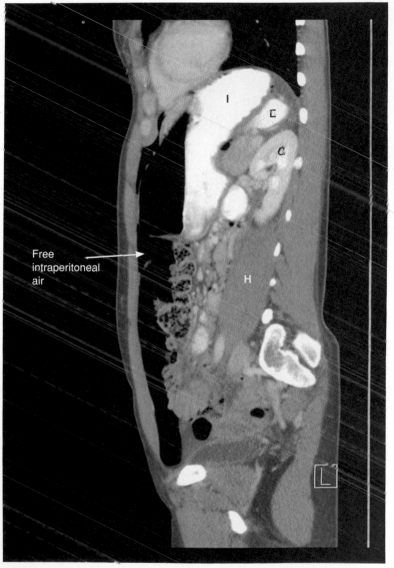

Free
intraperitoneal
air

FIGURE 3.6 E

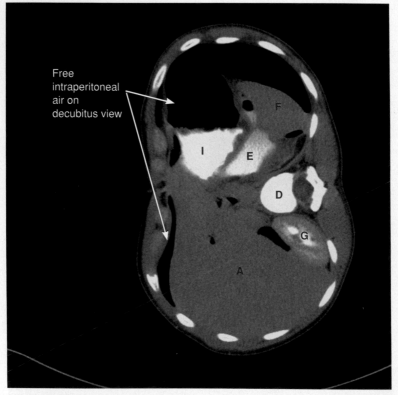

FIGURE 3.6 F

Duodenal Perforation

RADIOLOGY

- **Plain film/Upper GI findings**
  - Free air
  - Leak of contrast into the peritoneum
  - Mass effect onto the duodenum from an adjacent inflammatory reaction from the perforation can be seen
- **CT findings** (Fig. 3.7)
  - Free retroperitoneal air adjacent to the duodenum
  - Leak of oral contrast into the retroperitoneum
  - Duodenal wall edema
  - Peripancreatic fat stranding may be seen

FIGURE 3.7 A–C

A. Liver
B. Vertebra
C. Kidney
D. Renal vein
E. Descending aorta
F. IVC
G. Spleen

H. Small bowel loops
I. Bladder
J. Stomach
K. Pancreas
L. Superior mesenteric artery
M. Psoas muscle

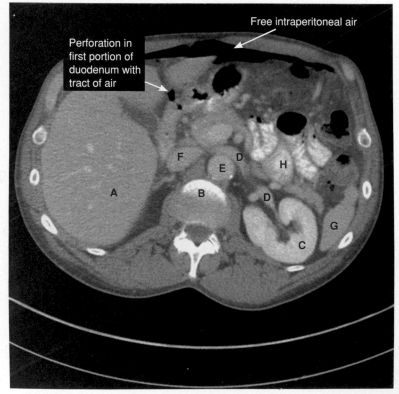

FIGURE 3.7 A

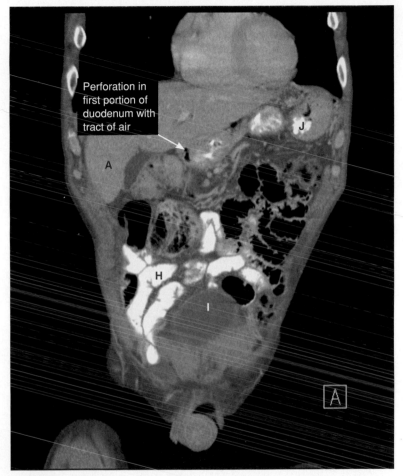

Perforation in first portion of duodenum with tract of air

FIGURE 3.7 B

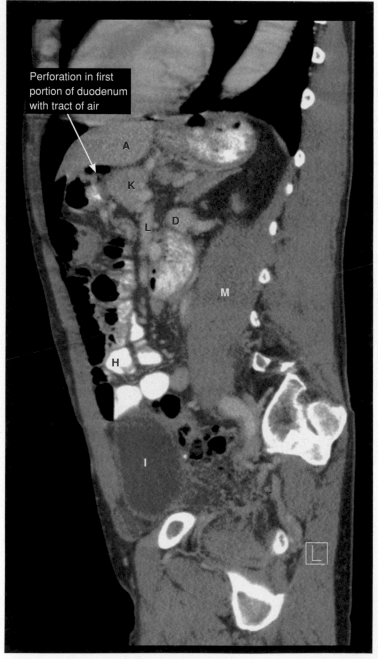

Perforation in first portion of duodenum with tract of air

FIGURE 3.7 C

Suggested Readings

Ba-Ssalamah A, Prokop M, Uffmann M, et al. Dedicated multidetector CT of the stomach: Spectrum of diseases. *Radiographics.* 2003;23:625–644.

Chen CY, Hsu JS, Wu DC, et al. Gastric cancer: Preoperative local staging with 3D multi-detector row CT–correlation with surgical and histopathologic results. *Radiology.* 2007;242:472–482.

Dempsey DT. Stomach. In: Charles Brunicardi F, et al., eds. *Schwartz's Principles of Surgery,* 9th ed. New York, NY: Mcgraw-Hill; Chapter 26. 2009.

Ghai S, Pattison J, Ghai S, et al. Primary gastrointestinal lymphoma: Spectrum of imaging findings with pathologic correlation. *Radiographics.* 2007;27:1371–1388.

Hayden CK Jr, Swischuk LE, Lobe TE, et al. Ultrasound: The definitive imaging modality in pyloric stenosis. *Radiographics.* 1984;4:517–530.

Hernanz-Schulman M. Infantile hypertrophic pyloric stenosis. *Radiology.* 2003;227: 319–331.

Iqbal CW, Rivard DC, Mortellaro VE, et al. Evaluation of ultrasonographic parameters in the diagnosis of pyloric stenosis relative to patient age and size. *J Pediatr Surg.* 2012;47(8):1542–1547.

Johnston FM, Varela JE, Hawkins WG. Stomach. In: Mary E. Klingensmith, et al., eds. *The Washington Manual of Surgery,* 6th ed. Philadelphia, PA: Lippincott Williams &Wilkins; Chapter 9. *J Natl Compr Canc Netw.* 2012;10:951–960.

Laine L, Jensen DM. Management of patients with ulcer bleeding. *Am J Gastroenterol.* 2012;107(3):345–360.

Levy AD, Remotti HE, Thompson WM, et al. Gastrointestinal stromal tumors: Radiologic features with pathologic correlation. *Radiographics.* 2003;23:283–304.

Lim JS, Yun MJ, Kim MJ, et al. CT and PET in stomach cancer: Preoperative staging and monitoring of response to therapy. *Radiographics.* 2006;26:143–156.

Low VH, Levine MS, Rubesin SE, et al. Diagnosis of gastric carcinoma: Sensitivity of double-contrast barium studies. *AJR Am J Roentgenol.* 1994;162:329–334.

Lunevicius R, Morkevicius M. Comparison of laparoscopic versus open repair for perforated duodenal ulcers. *Surg Endosc.* 2005;19(12):1565–1571.

Ly JQ. The Rigler sign. *Radiology.* 2003;228:706–707.

Merino S, Saiz A, Moreno MJ, et al. CT evaluation of gastric wall pathology. *Br J Radiol.* 1999;72:1124–1131.

Mitchell MT. Bariatric imaging: Technical aspects and postoperative complications. *Appl Radiol.* 2008;37(2):10–22.

Mitchell MT, Carabetta JM, Shah RN, et al. Duodenal switch gastric bypass surgery for morbid obesity: Imaging of postsurgical anatomy and postoperative gastrointestinal complications. *AJR Am J Roentgenol.* 2009;193(6):1576–1580.

Sato T, Sakai Y, Ishiguro S, et al. Radiologic manifestations of early gastric lymphoma. *AJR Am J Roentgenol.* 1986;146:513–517.

Siddiqui S, Heidel RE, Angel CA, et al. Pyloromyotomy: Randomized control trial of laparoscopic vs open technique. *J Pediatr Surg.* 2012;47(1):93–98.

Zissin R, Osadchy A, Gayer G. Abdominal CT findings in small bowel perforation. *Br J Radiol.* 2009;82:162–171.

Gallbladder

Gallbladder Disease

Overview

- Cholesterol gallstones (85%) are the most common
  - Risk factors: Four Fs (female, fertile, fat, and forty)
  - Due to imbalance between bile, lecithin, and cholesterol
- Pigmented stones (15%)
  - Risk factors: Hemolytic disorders, biliary tract infection, ileal resection, cirrhosis

Definitions

Acute cholecystitis—inflammation of the gallbladder from stone impaction in the cystic duct

Choledocholithiasis—gallstone in the common bile duct which may lead to cholangitis

Signs and Symptoms

- Acute cholecystitis—leukocytosis and right upper quadrant pain
  - Murphy's sign: Deep palpation of the liver edge during inspiratory phase worsens the pain, causing patient to cease inspiration
- Choledocholithiasis/ascending cholangitis
  - Charcot's triad: Fever, jaundice, and right upper quadrant pain
  - Reynold's pentad: Charcot's triad + altered mental status + shock

Diagnosis

- Ultrasound is the test of choice with high sensitivity and specificity
  - Acute cholecystitis
    - Gallbladder wall thickening (greater than 3 mm), gallbladder distension (greater than 10 × 4 cm), pericholecystic fluid, gallstone impacted in the cystic duct, and sonographic Murphy's sign (Murphy's sign pressing the ultrasound probe over the visualized gallbladder).
    - Evaluate common bile duct size to determine if there is dilatation and/or choledocholithiasis
  - HIDA scan can be helpful if findings are not definitive on ultrasound
    - Non-visualization of the gallbladder even after administering morphine (which closes the Sphincter of Oddi)

Treatment

- Symptomatic cholelithiasis, biliary dyskinesia—elective laparoscopic cholecystectomy
- Acute cholecystitis—antibiotics, laparoscopic cholecystectomy
  - Percutaneous cholecystostomy tube for ICU patients or patients who cannot tolerate surgery
- Choledocholithiasis, ascending cholangitis—endoscopic retrograde cholangiopancreatography (ERCP)
  - Percutaneous transhepatic tube placement if ERCP is not available or if patient's anatomy does not allow for ERCP
- Indications for intraoperative cholangiogram
  - Previous history of choledocholithiasis, elevated liver function tests, gallstone pancreatitis
  - Ultrasound showing dilated biliary duct
  - Uncertainty of the anatomy during cholecystectomy

Other Important Facts

- Gallbladder wall calcification (porcelain gallbladder)—Perform cholecystectomy due to increased risk of gallbladder cancer
- Gallbladder polyp—Perform cholecystectomy for patients who are symptomatic, polyps >1 cm, in patients greater than 50 years old, fast-growing/sessile polyps

- Be mindful of gallbladder adenocarcinoma presenting acutely. Look for signs of an invasive gallbladder fossa mass, liver invasion or metastases, and lymphadenopathy.

RADIOLOGY

Acute Cholecystitis

- **US findings** (Fig. 4.1)
  - Gallbladder distention with dimensions greater than 10 × 4 cm
  - Pericholecystic fluid
  - Gallbladder wall thickening greater than 3 mm
  - Positive sonographic Murphy's sign (the most specific finding)
- **CT findings**
  - Gallbladder wall thickening and distention
  - Pericholecystic fluid
  - Fat stranding around gallbladder
  - Gallstones are seen in minority of cases as either high- or low-density masses
- **HIDA findings**
  - Nonvisualization of gallbladder resulting from cystic duct obstruction
  - Imaging performed 2 to 4 hours after administration of tracer, sometimes with the administration of morphine (which closes the Sphincter of Oddi to improve sensitivity)

FIGURE 4.1 A,B

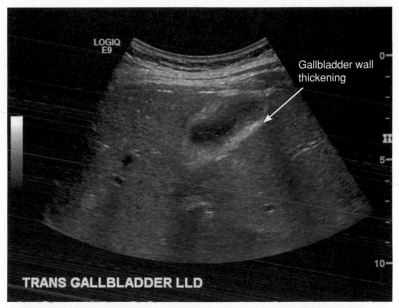

FIGURE 4.1 A

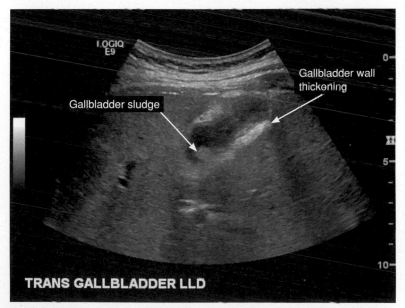

FIGURE 4.1 B

Cholelithiasis

- **Plain film findings**
  - Only 10% to 15% of gallstones are radiopaque
- **US findings** (Fig. 4.2)
  - Most accurate in detecting gallstones; sensitivity is greater than 95%
  - Appear as echogenic foci with or without posterior acoustic clean shadowing—which are black (not gray) lines extending away from the transducer from the stone
  - Gallbladder full of stones may show a "wall-echo-shadow" complex characterized by two parallel curved echogenic lines separated by thin anechoic stripe with dense posterior acoustic shadowing distal to the deeper echogenic line
  - Not to be confused with gallbladder sludge which are more amorphous and less echogenic than stones
- **CT findings** (Fig. 4.3)
  - Minority of stones are visible
  - May be hyper- or hypodense, or of mixed density

FIGURE 4.2 A–D

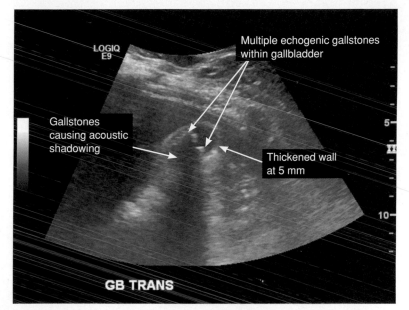

FIGURE 4.2 A

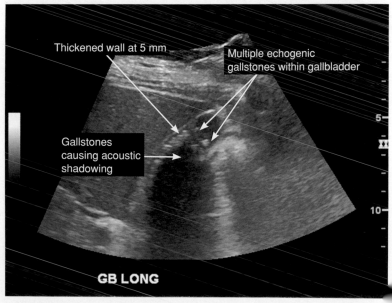

FIGURE 4.2 B

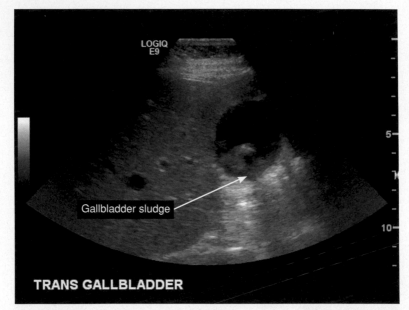

FIGURE 4.2 C

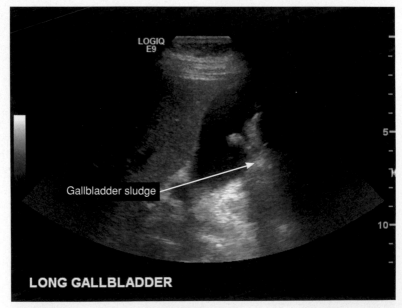

FIGURE 4.2 D

FIGURE 4.3 A–C

A. Liver
B. Kidney
C. Psoas muscle

D. Vertebra
E. Small bowel loops
F. Bladder

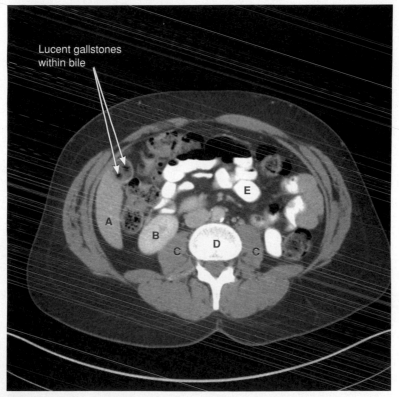

FIGURE 4.3 A

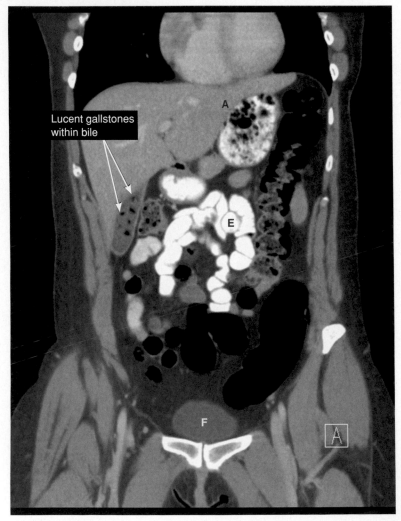

FIGURE 4.3 B

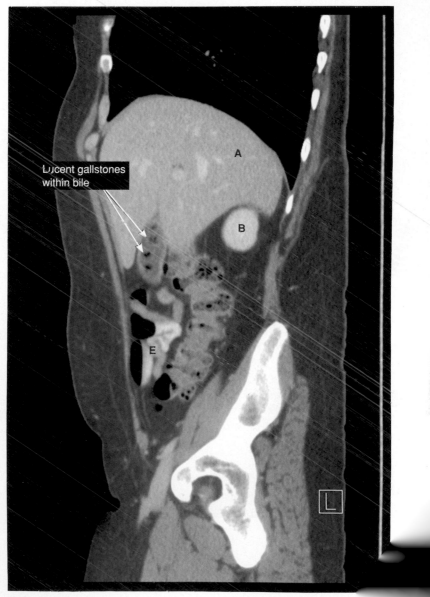

Lucent gallstones
within bile

A

B

E

FIGURE 4.3 C

Emphysematous Gallbladder

- **Plain film findings**
  - Intramural or intraluminal gas seen in the RUQ
- **US findings** (Fig. 4.4)
  - Curvilinear, bright echogenic reflectors with dirty shadowing—which are gray (not black), hazy lines extending away from the transducer to the inferior edge of the screen
- **CT findings** (Fig. 4.5)
  - Intramural and intraluminal gas are noted in the gallbladder

FIGURE 4.4 A–C

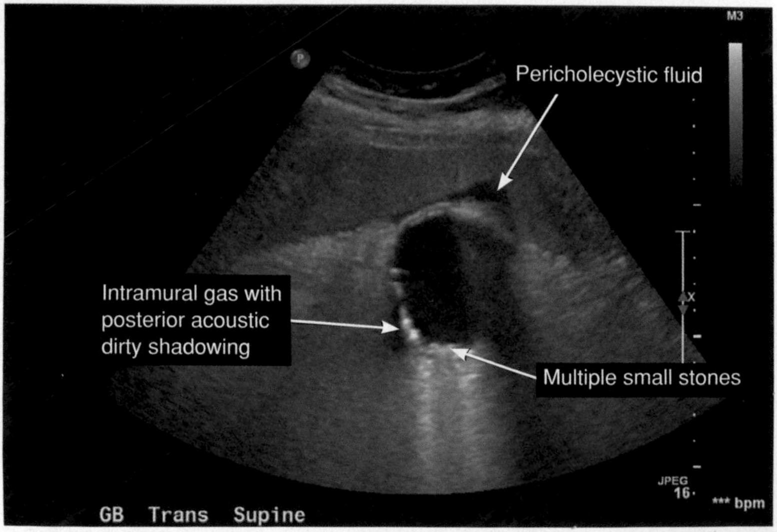

Pericholecystic fluid

Intramural gas with posterior acoustic dirty shadowing

Multiple small stones

GB Trans Supine

FIGURE 4.4 A

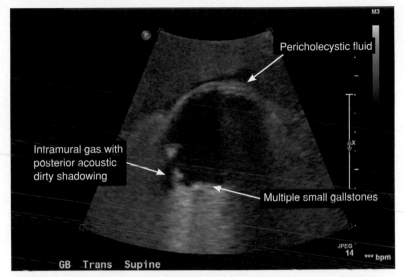

FIGURE 4.4 B

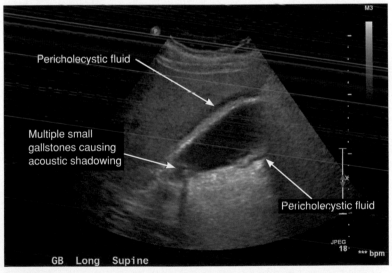

FIGURE 4.4 C

FIGURE 4.5 A–C

A. Liver

B. Small bowel loops

C. Vertebra

D. Stomach

E. Kidney

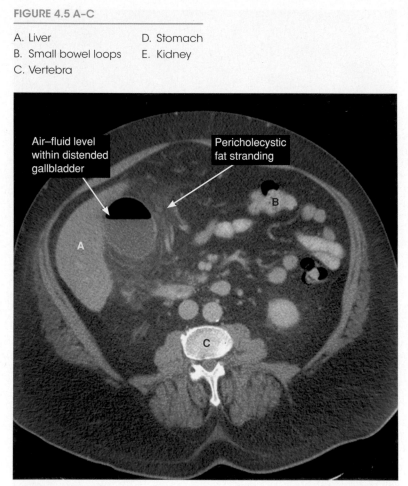

Air–fluid level within distended gallbladder

Pericholecystic fat stranding

FIGURE 4.5 A

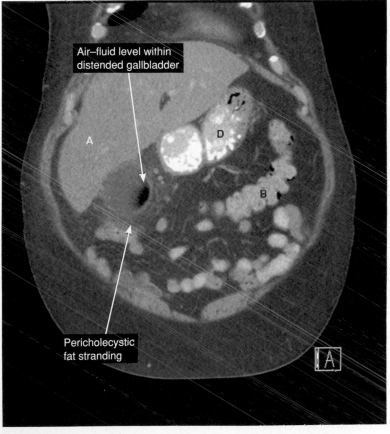

FIGURE 4.5 B

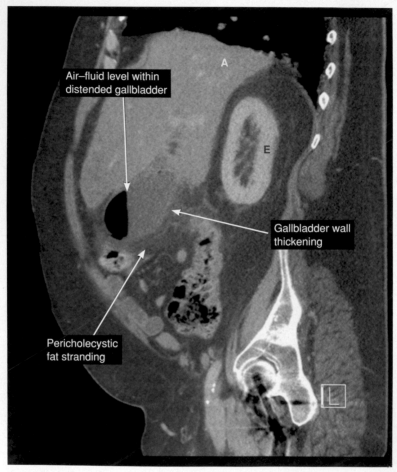

FIGURE 4.5 C

Gallbladder Calcification

- **Plain film findings**
  - Dense calcifications in the RUQ
- **US findings**
  - Bright echogenic reflectors with clean (black) posterior acoustic shadowing
  - The posterior wall of the gallbladder is visible, unlike in a "wall-echo-shadow" complex, which obscures the posterior wall
- **CT findings** (Fig. 4.6)
  - Calcification noted along the walls of the gallbladder

FIGURE 4.6 A,B

A. Liver	C. Kidney
B. Small bowel loops	D. Vertebra

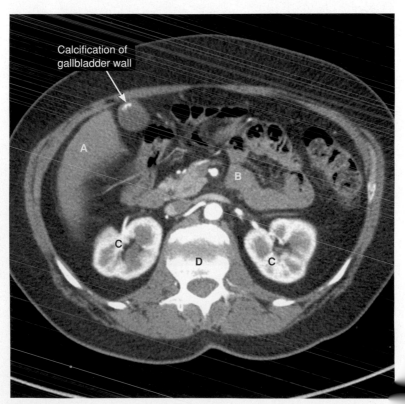

Calcification of gallbladder wall

FIGURE 4.6 A

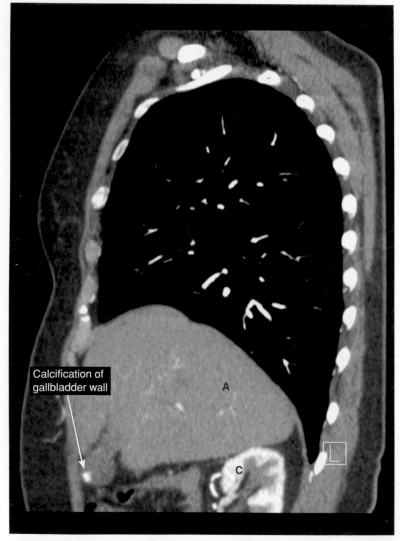

Calcification of gallbladder wall

FIGURE 4.6 B

Gallbladder Polyp

- **US findings** (Fig. 4.7)
  - Cholesterol polyps are noted as small, nonmobile (unlike gallstones), echogenic masses usually less than 5 mm
  - Adenomatous polyps seen as echogenic masses larger than 10 mm
- **CT findings**
  - Cholesterol polyps are benign masses found in 5% of the population usually measuring less than 5 mm, usually not visible on CT
  - Adenomatous polyps are masses measuring larger than 10 mm with premalignant potential

FIGURE 4.7 A,B

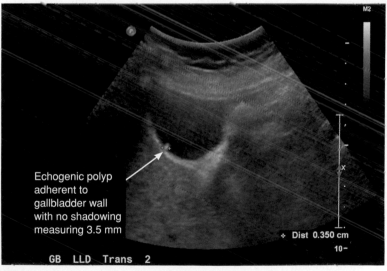

Echogenic polyp adherent to gallbladder wall with no shadowing measuring 3.5 mm

✢ Dist 0.350 cm

GB   LLD   Trans   2

FIGURE 4.7 A

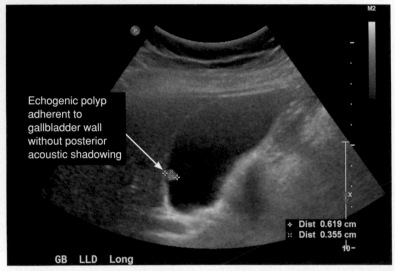

Echogenic polyp adherent to gallbladder wall without posterior acoustic shadowing

FIGURE 4.7 B

Choledocholithiasis

- Intraoperative cholangiogram (Fig. 4.8)
- **US findings**
  - If obstructive, proximal intra- and/or extra-hepatic bile duct dilation will be seen
- **CT findings**
  - Radiopaque stone surrounded by lower-density bile within the intra- or extra-hepatic bile ducts
  - If obstructive, proximal bile duct dilation can be seen
- **MRCP findings**
  - Intraductal signal voids are noted with or without proximal bile duct dilation
  - Gas bubbles, intraductal masses, or blood clots may cause false positives

FIGURE 4.8 A,B

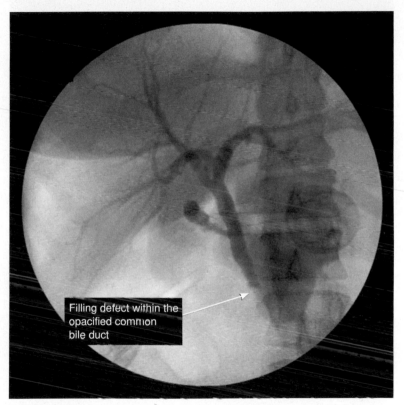

Filling defect within the opacified common bile duct

FIGURE 4.8 A

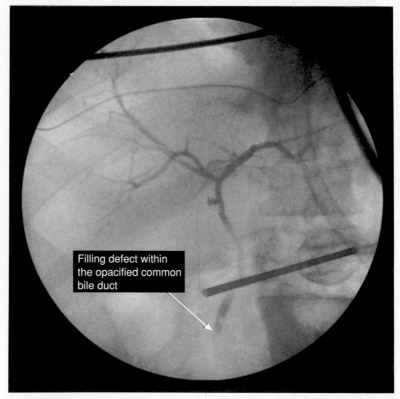

Filling defect within the opacified common bile duct

FIGURE 4.8 B

Suggested Readings

Anderson SW, Lucey BC, Borghese JC, et al. Accuracy of MDCT in the diagnosis of choledocholithiasis. *AJR Am J Roentgenol*. 2006;187:174–180.

Andrén-Sandberg A. Diagnosis and management of gallbladder polyps. *N Am J Med Sci*. 2012;4(5):203–211.

Bortoff GA, Chen MY, Ott DJ, et al. Gallbladder stones: Imaging and intervention. *Radiographics*. 2000;20:751–766.

Corwin MT, Siewert B, Sheiman RG, et al. Incidentally detected gallbladder polyps: Is follow-up necessary? – Long-term clinical and US analysis of 346 patients. *Radiology*. 2011;258:277–282.

Grayson DE, Abbott RM, Levy AD, et al. Emphysematous infections of the abdomen and pelvis: A pictorial review. *Radiographics*. 2002;22:543–561.

Levy AD, Murakata LA, Rohrmann CA Jr. Gallbladder carcinoma: Radiologic pathologic correlation. *Radiographics*. 2001;21:295–314.

O'Connor OJ, Maher MM. Imaging of cholecystitis. *AJR Am J Roentgenol*. 2011; 196:W367–W374.

Soto JA, Barish MA, Alvarez O, et al. Detection of choledocholithiasis with MR cholangiography: Comparison of three-dimensional fast spin-echo and single- and multisection half-Fourier rapid acquisition with relaxation enhancement sequences. *Radiology*. 2000;215:737–745.

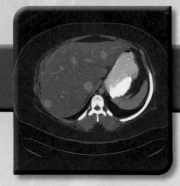

Liver

Pyogenic Abscess

- Spread via:
  - Biliary system (obstruction)
    - Most common
    - For example: cholangiocarcinoma, CBD stone
  - Hematogenous spread
    - For example: appendicitis, diverticulitis
- Single abscess or multiple abscesses
- More common in the right hepatic lobe
- Bacteria
  - Monomicrobial 40%, polymicrobial 40%, culture negative 20%
  - Gram-negative organisms most common
  - *Escherichia coli* found in two-thirds of abscesses
  - Opportunistic organisms in AIDS patients
    - Fungal and mycobacterial
  - Blood cultures positive, ~50% of cases
- Presenting signs and symptoms
  - Fever (most common), right upper quadrant abdominal pain/tenderness, jaundice
- Treatment
  - Antibiotics and drainage
  - Manage etiology of the pyogenic abscess

Amebic Abscess

- Caused by *Entamoeba histolytica*
- Most common abscess worldwide—infects up to 10% of worldwide population
- Amebic cysts are ingested, passing through stomach and small bowel unharmed → trophozoite in colon → spreads into liver via portal venous system from colon
- Presenting signs and symptoms
  - History of recent travel to endemic areas
  - Right upper quadrant pain, fever, jaundice, diarrhea
  - Labs
    - Serologic testing
    - Leukocytosis
    - Normal bilirubin
- Treatment
  - Metronidazole

RADIOLOGY

General Liver Abscess (Fig. 5.1)

- Multilocular, rim enhancing mass with focal areas of fluid attenuation representing blood or pus

FIGURE 5.1 A,B

A. Heart   D. Spleen
B. Vertebra   E. Descending aorta
C. Kidney

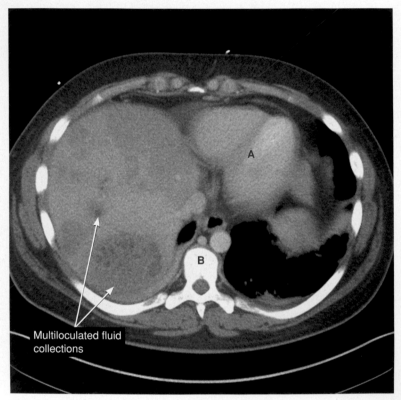

FIGURE 5.1 A

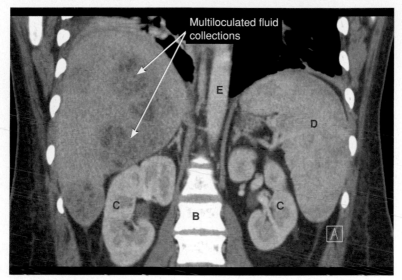

Multiloculated fluid collections

FIGURE 5.1 B

Pyogenic Abscess

- **Chest x-ray**
  - Nonspecific findings—elevated right hemidiaphragm, right-sided pleural effusion, and atelectasis can be seen
- **Ultrasound**
  - Multiloculated fluid collection within the liver, sometimes with posterior acoustic enhancement
- **CT findings**
  - Multilocular fluid collection ± air–fluid levels with areas of peripheral enhancement

Amebic Abscess

- **Ultrasound**
  - Typically, a round hypoechoic, homogeneous lesion with posterior acoustic enhancement
- **CT findings**
  - Round, rim-enhancing hypodense lesions with a peripheral zone of edema
  - May contain central septations

Hemangioma

- Most common benign tumor of the liver
- More common in females (3:1)
- If greater than 5 cm then considered a giant hemangioma
- Mostly asymptomatic. Normal LFTs and tumor markers
- If symptomatic: Kasabach–Merritt syndrome (presents with bruising, purpura, thrombocytopenia with consumptive coagulopathy, microangiopathic hemolytic anemia)
- Treatment
  - Surgical resection if ruptured, significant change in size, development of Kasabach–Merritt syndrome

RADIOLOGY

- **CT findings** (Fig. 5.2)
  - Relatively hypodense and well-defined lesion when compared to surrounding liver in precontrast phase
  - Early peripheral nodular enhancement, with enhancement equivalent to blood pool
  - Centripetal contrast enhancement on more delayed images
- **MRI findings**
  - T1-weighted images may show low signal intensity
  - T2-weighted images show high signal intensity
  - Peripheral enhancement with equivalent signal intensity to aorta on arterial phase, with centripetal enhancement on more delayed phases

FIGURE 5.2 A,B

A. Stomach
B. Small bowel loops
C. Vertebra

D. Kidney
E. Spleen

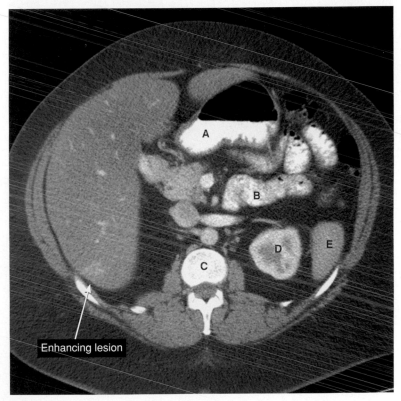

FIGURE 5.2 A

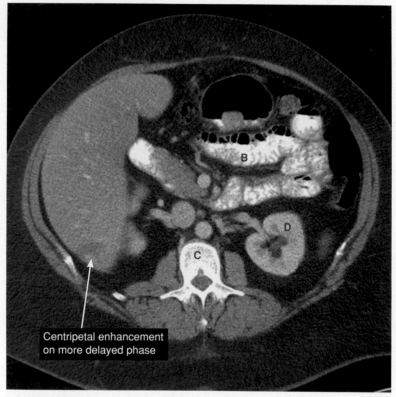

Centripetal enhancement on more delayed phase

FIGURE 5.2 B

Focal Nodular Hyperplasia

- Cord of benign hepatocytes
- Second most common benign tumor of the liver
- Unlikely to rupture
- Possibly related to vascular malformation

RADIOLOGY

- **CT findings** (Fig. 5.3)
  - Iso- to hyper-dense mass classically with a central, spoke-wheel appearing scar
  - Increased arterial enhancement with respect to the normal liver parenchyma which equilibrates with normal liver on portal venous phases, and retains contrast on more delayed images
  - Central scar classically enhances on delayed images
- **MRI findings**
  - Best evaluated with a hepatobiliary gadolinium contrast agent
  - Same enhancement pattern as described above
  - Central scar will be hyperintense on T2-weighted images

FIGURE 5.3 A–F

A. Stomach   E. Portal vein
B. Descending aorta F. Pancreas
C. Vertebra   G. Small bowel loops
D. Spleen   H. IVC

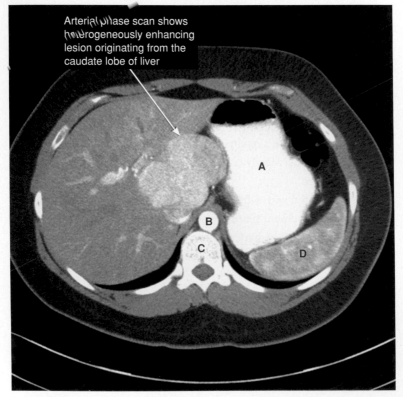

Arterial phase scan shows heterogeneously enhancing lesion originating from the caudate lobe of liver

FIGURE 5.3 A

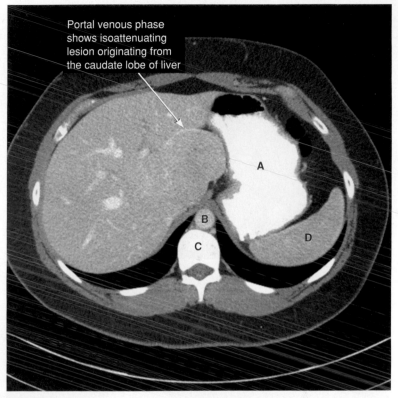

FIGURE 5.3 B

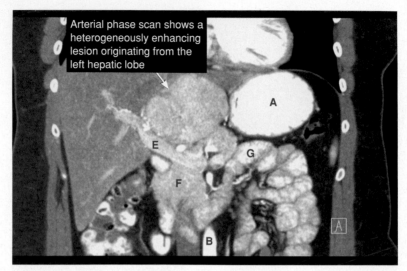

FIGURE 5.3 C

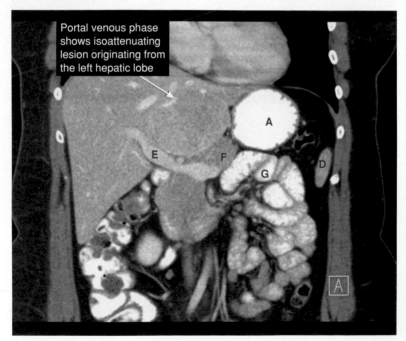

FIGURE 5.3 D

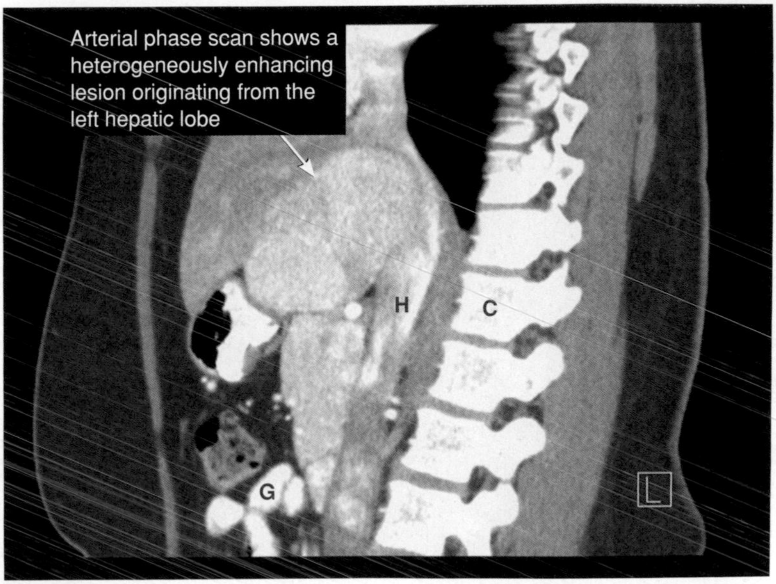

Arterial phase scan shows a heterogeneously enhancing lesion originating from the left hepatic lobe

H   C

G

L

FIGURE 5.3 E

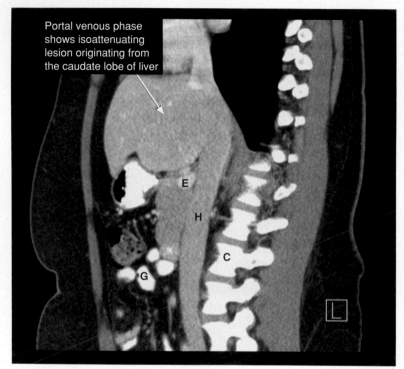

Portal venous phase shows isoattenuating lesion originating from the caudate lobe of liver

E

H

C

G

L

FIGURE 5.3 F

Hepatic Adenoma

- Benign proliferation of hepatocytes
- More common in females, associated with oral contraceptives
- Greater than 10 lesions = adenomatosis
- Risk of hemorrhagic rupture and malignant transformation

RADIOLOGY

- **CT findings** (Fig. 5.4)
  - Typically solitary, although multiple lesions can be present
  - Lobular mass sometimes associated with hemorrhage
  - Usually demonstrates heterogeneous enhancement

- **MRI findings**
  - On T1-weighted images, appear hyperintense (usually indicating hemorrhage) or isointense
  - On T2-weighted images, heterogeneously hyperintense
  - Often have a fatty component, best seen on in and opposed-phase imaging

FIGURE 5.4 A,B

A. Stomach   D. Small bowel loops
B. Spleen   E. IVC
C. Vertebra

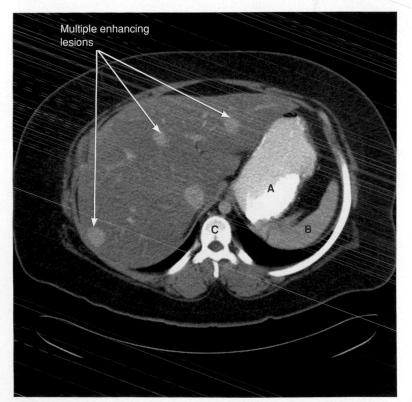

FIGURE 5.4 A

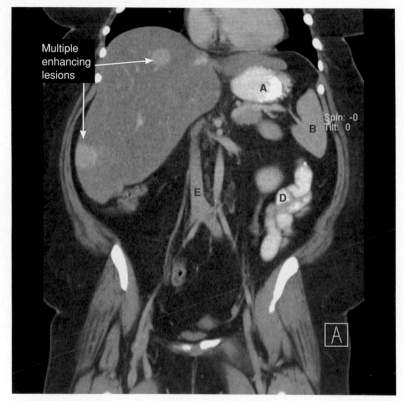

FIGURE 5.4 B

Hepatocellular Carcinoma

- Most common primary malignancy of liver
- 75% related to chronic HBV and HCV infection (worldwide HBV more common)
- **Risk factors**
  - Cirrhosis, smoking, EtOH, HBV/HCV infection
- **Signs and symptoms**
  - Usually asymptomatic until late
  - Vague right upper quadrant pain radiating to shoulder
  - Hepatic decompensation in patient with mild cirrhosis
    Rarely rupture (sudden pain followed by hypovolemic shock)

- **Labs**
  - Elevated alpha-fetoprotein (>200 ng/mL in 75% of cases)
- **Treatment**
  - Liver transplant
  - Surgical resection
  - Radiofrequency ablation
  - Transcatheter arterial chemoembolization

RADIOLOGY

- **Ultrasound** (Fig. 5.5A)
  - Useful screening tool for cirrhotic patients
  - Solid mass of variable echogenicity
- **CT findings** (Fig. 5.5B,C)
  - Often seen in the background of a shrunken, nodular, cirrhotic liver
  - Classically, enhances more than liver parenchyma on the arterial phase, and washes out on delayed phases
  - May be associated with transient hepatic attenuation difference, arterioportal shunting, and invasion of the portal veins
- **MRI findings** (Fig. 5.5 D–F)
  - Very useful screening tool for patients at high risk
  - Arterially enhancing lesion which washes out on delayed images on dynamic contrast images, often in the background of a cirrhotic liver
  - May contain intratumoral microscopic fat, best seen on in and opposed phase images
  - Usually T2 hyperintense
  - May be associated with portal vein thrombosis
  - Fibrolamellar HCC subtype seen in younger patients without cirrhosis
    - Usually heterogeneous enhancement on arterial phase
    - May be associated with a central scar that is T2 hypointense (unlike focal nodular hyperplasia) and contains calcifications

FIGURE 5.5 A–C

A. Stomach   E. IVC
B. Spleen   F. Kidney
C. Vertebra   G. Psoas muscle
D. Descending aorta

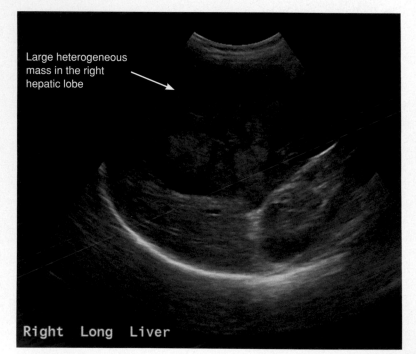

FIGURE 5.5 A

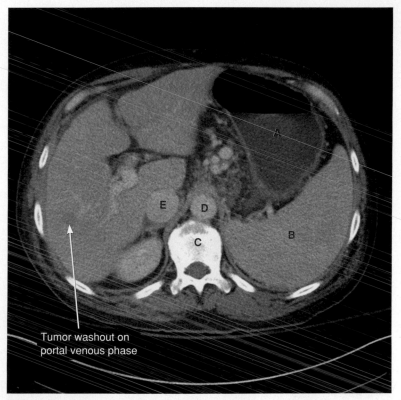

Tumor washout on
portal venous phase

FIGURE 5.5 B

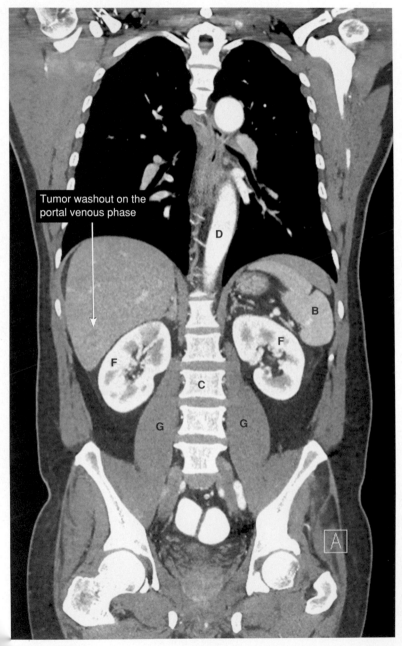

Tumor washout on the portal venous phase

FIGURE 5.5 C

FIGURE 5.5 D–F

A. Kidney D. Vertebra
B. IVC E. Pancreas
C. Descending aorta F. Spleen

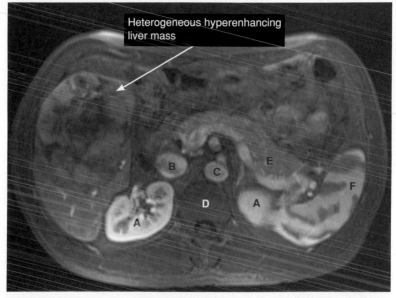

FIGURE 5.5 D

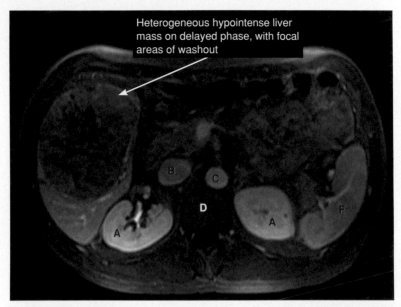

FIGURE 5.5 E

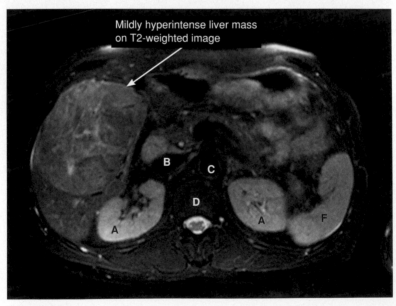

FIGURE 5.5 F

Pneumobilia

- Etiology
  - Biliary-enteric surgical anastomosis
  - Biliary-enteric fistula
  - Incompetent sphincter of Oddi, for example: post ERCP
  - Infection (rare), for example: emphysematous cholecystitis, cholangitis

RADIOLOGY

- **Ultrasound**
  - Bright echogenic foci within the bile ducts with echogenic lines extending away from the transducer (reverberation artifact)
- **CT findings** (Fig. 5.6)
  - Gas located near the liver hilum (unlike portal venous gas which travels towards the liver periphery)
  - Predilection for left lobe due to the more ventral location compared to the right lobe of liver

FIGURE 5.6 A,B

A. Stomach   E. Spleen
B. IVC   F. Small bowel loops
C. Descending aorta   G. Portal vein
D. Vertebra

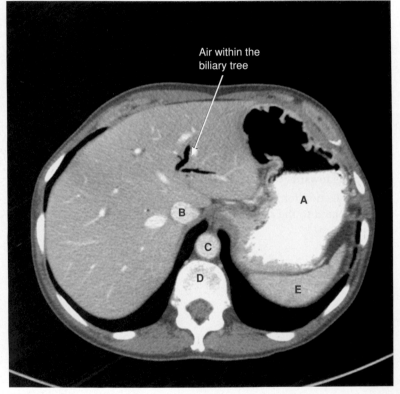

FIGURE 5.6 A

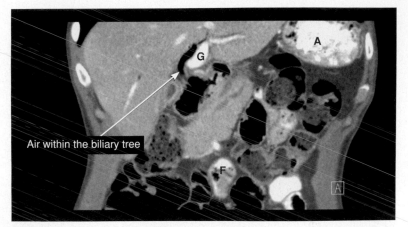

FIGURE 5.6 B

Portal Vein Thrombosis

- **CT findings** (Fig. 5.7)
  - Nonenhancing filling defect within the lumen of the portal veins on contrast enhanced images
  - Tumor thrombus enhances and may expand the portal veins
  - The hepatic segment supplied by the occluded portal vein will demonstrate transient hepatic attenuation difference (phenomenon where the affected liver segment is higher in attenuation than the rest of the liver)

FIGURE 5.7 A–C

A. Liver
B. Stomach
C. Spleen
D. Descending aorta

E. IVC
F. Vertebra
G. Peritoneal free fluid
H. Kidney

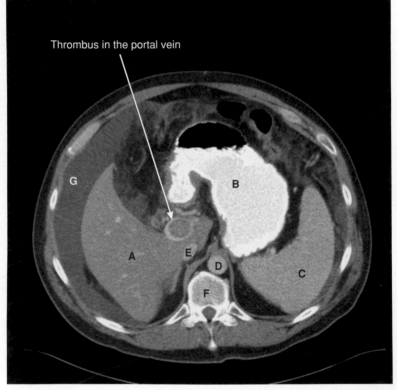

Thrombus in the portal vein

FIGURE 5.7 A

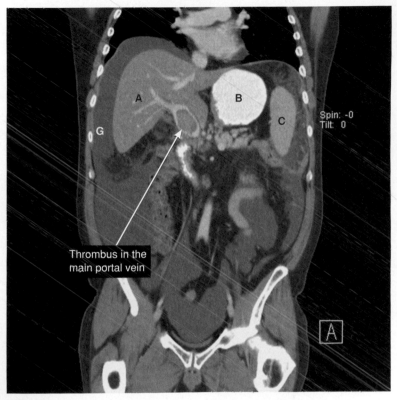

FIGURE 5.7 B

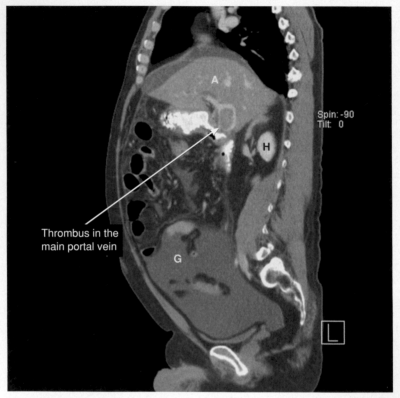

FIGURE 5.7 C

Suggested Readings

Brancatelli G, Federie MP, Grazioli L, et al. Focal nodular hyperplasia: CT findings with emphasis on multiphasic helical CT in 78 patients. *Radiology.* 2001;219:61–68.

Clark HP, Carson WF, Kavanagh PV, et al. Staging and current treatment of hepatocellular carcinoma. *Radiographics.* 2005;25:S3–S23.

Gabata T, Kadoya M, Matsui O, et al. Dynamic CT of hepatic abscesses: Significance of transient segmental enhancement. *AJR Am J Roentgenol.* 2001;176:675–679.

Grazioli L, Federie MP, Brancatelli G, et al. Hepatic adenomas: Imaging and pathologic findings. *Radiographics.* 2001;21:877–894.

Horton KM, Bluemke DA, Hruban RH, et al. CT and MR imaging of benign hepatic and biliary tumors. *Radiographics.* 1999;19:431–451.

Mori R, Raval B, Sandler CM. Portal vein thrombosis: Imaging findings. *AJR Am J Roentgenol.* 1994;162:77–81.

Sebastia C, Quiroga S, Espin E, et al. Portomesenteric vein gas: Pathologic mechanism, findings, and prognosis. *Radiographics.* 2000;20:1213–1224.

Hussain HK, Adusumilli S, et al. MR imaging of hepatocellular carcinoma in the cirrhotic liver: Challenges and controversies. *Radiology.* 2008;247:311–330.

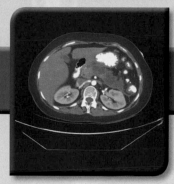

Pancreas

Acute Pancreatitis

Overview

- The two most common causes are gallstones and alcohol
- Other etiologies include iatrogenic (endoscopic retrograde cholangiopancreatography [ERCP]), drugs, trauma, neoplasm, hypercalcemia, hypertriglyceridemia, infections, idiopathic

Signs and Symptoms

- Epigastric pain radiating to the back accompanied with nausea and vomiting
- May develop classic signs of Grey Turner's sign (flank ecchymosis) or Cullen's sign (periumbilical ecchymosis); suggests hemorrhagic pancreatitis
- Pancreatitis may lead to acute respiratory distress syndrome (ARDS) or systemic inflammatory response (SIRS) with resultant hypotension, tachycardia, tachypnea, etc.

Diagnosis

- Elevated amylase and lipase—no correlation between the serum level and the prognosis or the severity of the disease process
- Ranson's criteria:
  - Upon admission:
    - Age >55 years
    - White blood cell count >16,000 cells/mm³

- ◦ Glucose >200 mg/dL
- ◦ Serum lactate dehydrogenase >350 IU/L
- ◦ Aspartate aminotransferase >250 IU/L
- At 48 hours:
  - ◦ Hematocrit decrease >10%
  - ◦ Blood urea nitrogen elevation >5 mg/dL
  - ◦ Calcium <8 mg/dL
  - ◦ Arterial PO_2 <60 mmHg
  - ◦ Base deficit >4 mEq/L
  - ◦ Estimated fluid sequestration >6 L
- Number of Ranson's signs: Risk of mortality
  0–2: 0%
  3–4: 15%
  5–6: 50%
  >6: 70%–90%

Complications

- Pancreatic pseudocyst
- Necrotizing pancreatitis
- Infected pancreatic necrosis
- Visceral pseudoaneurysm

Treatment

- Supportive measures: IV fluid resuscitation, bowel rest to limit pancreatic enzyme secretions, TPN or postpyloric nasojejunal feeding, pain control, alcohol withdrawal prophylaxis, antibiotics for infected or necrotizing pancreatitis
- If pancreatitis is caused by gallstones, then patient should undergo a semielective cholecystectomy with intraoperative cholangiogram during the same hospitalization
- Surgical treatment is usually reserved for patients with infected or necrotizing pancreatitis who are not improving despite maximal medical management
  - Involves necrosectomy, drain placement, and possible serial abdominal washouts

RADIOLOGY

Pancreatitis with Surrounding Fluid

- **Plain film findings**
  - Duodenal ileus may be seen
  - Sentinel dilated loop of transverse colon can be seen with acute pancreatitis
  - Effacement of the psoas fat plane
  - Chronic pancreatitis may show pancreatic calcifications
- **US findings**
  - Chronic pancreatitis shows main pancreatic duct dilatation beyond the normal 3 mm
  - Acute pancreatitis will manifest as a diffuse or focal hypoechogenicity of the pancreas with or without surrounding peripancreatic fluid
- **CT findings** (Fig. 6.1)
  - Diffuse or focal pancreatic edema with peripancreatic fat stranding
  - May be associated with surrounding fluid collections
  - Areas of non-enhancement of the pancreas would be concerning for necrotizing pancreatitis
  - Areas of high attenuation fluid within the pancreas would be concerning for hemorrhagic pancreatitis
  - May see associated complications including pseudocyst, splenic vein thrombosis, or splenic artery pseudoaneurysm
- **MRCP findings**
  - Chronic pancreatitis is characterized by dilatation or multifocal stenosis of main pancreatic duct sometimes with narrowing of the intrapancreatic segment of the common bile duct
  - Acute pancreatitis may manifest as a diffuse or focal T2 hyperintense signal within and/or surrounding the pancreas

FIGURE 6.1

A. Liver   D. Descending aorta
B. Kidney   E. Spleen
C. Vertebra

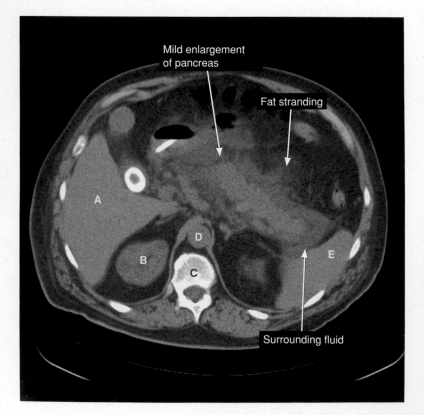

Pancreatitis with Necrosis

- **CT findings** (Fig. 6.2)
  - Areas of nonenhancement seen within pancreatic parenchyma in the setting of acute pancreatitis
  - Presence of air bubbles within loculated areas of necrotic tissue and fluid is highly suggestive of infection

FIGURE 6.2 A,B

A. Liver   D. Small bowel loops
B. Kidney   E. Stomach
C. Vertebra

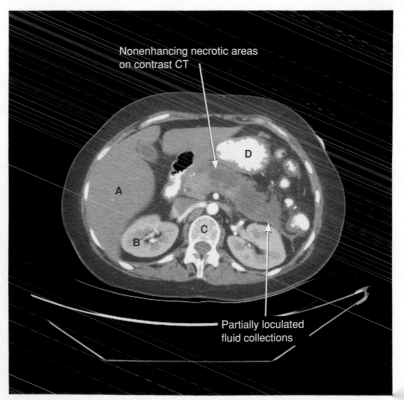

Nonenhancing necrotic areas on contrast CT

Partially loculated fluid collections

FIGURE 6.2 A

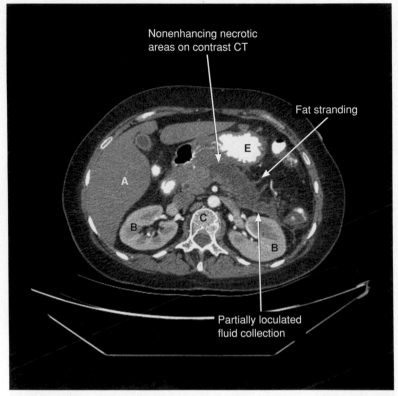

Nonenhancing necrotic
areas on contrast CT

Fat stranding

E

A

B

C

B

Partially loculated
fluid collection

FIGURE 6.2 B

Pseudocyst

Overview

- Defined as a peripancreatic fluid collection without epithelial lining
- Approximately 25% of acute pancreatitis will have acute pancreatic fluid collection
- If the acute pancreatic fluid collection persists longer than 4 to 6 weeks, it is defined as a pancreatic pseudocyst

Clinical Presentation

- Upper abdominal pain, symptoms from compression of adjacent viscera (early satiety, weight loss, nausea, vomiting, jaundice)

Complications

- Infected pseudocyst
- Obstruction of adjacent viscera (gastric outlet obstruction, biliary obstruction, hydronephrosis, etc.)
- Hemorrhage as a result of erosion into surrounding visceral vessels
- Rupture

Diagnosis

- CT, MR, or ultrasound
  - Pseudocysts <4 cm usually resolve spontaneously

Treatment

- Observation: If patient is asymptomatic, pseudocyst <6 cm in size
- Cystoenteric drainage
  - Endoscopic cystogastrostomy
  - Open or laparoscopic cystogastrostomy, cystoduodenostomy, or cystojejunostomy based on patient's anatomy

---

KEY POINT

- Biopsy of the cyst wall should always be obtained to rule out cystic neoplasm

RADIOLOGY

- **CT findings** (Fig. 6.3)
  - Homogeneous fluid collection persisting for greater than 4 weeks after an acute pancreatitis episode
  - Well-defined fluid collection with a thin capsule

FIGURE 6.3 A–C

A. Liver	E. Small bowel loops
B. Kidney	F. Stomach
C. Descending aorta	G. Spleen
D. Vertebra	

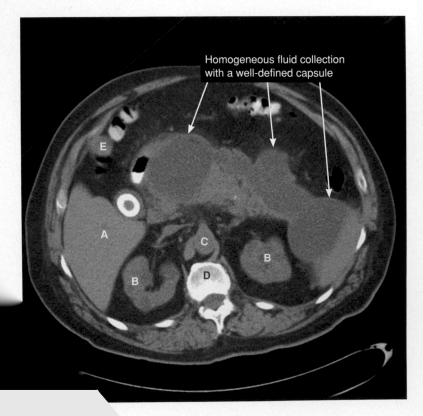

Homogeneous fluid collection with a well-defined capsule

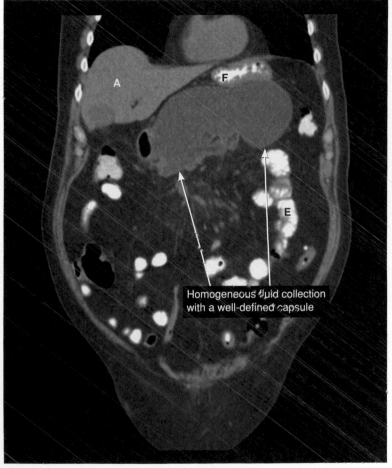

Homogeneous fluid collection
with a well-defined capsule

FIGURE 6.3 B

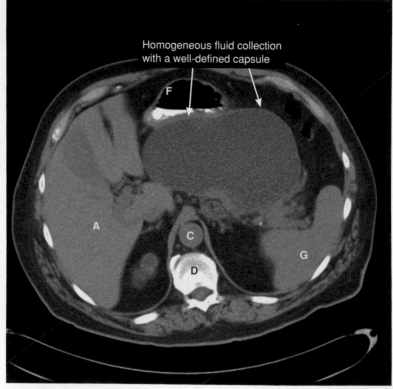

Homogeneous fluid collection with a well-defined capsule

FIGURE 6.3 C

Pancreatic Tumors and Cystic Diseases of the Pancreas

Overview

- Pancreatic cancer: 90% are ductal adenocarcinoma
- Poor prognosis: 5% 5-year survival, 20% if resectable
- Location: 70% occurs at the head, 20% in the body, 10% in the tail of the pancreas

Risk Factors

- Smoking
- Alcoholism
- Chronic pancreatitis
- Family history

Clinical Presentation

- Midepigastric pain, weight loss, painless jaundice, malaise
- Elevated CA19-9
- Courvoisier's sign: Painless jaundice with a palpable gallbladder
- Trousseau's sign: Migratory thrombophlebitis

KEY POINTS

- Radiologic imaging helps determine whether a tumor is resectable or not
  - Evaluate the anatomical relationship between the tumor and the superior mesenteric vein (SMV), portal vein, superior mesenteric artery (SMA), gastroduodenal artery (GDA), hepatic artery, and celiac artery
  - Considered nonresectable if there is distant metastasis, venous thrombosis of the SMV or portal vein, invasion of the SMA, hepatic artery, or celiac vessels

Pancreatic Cystic Lesions

Serous cystadenoma:

- Considered benign and usually asymptomatic. More commonly found in the head of the pancreas
  - Classic CT finding: Multilocular, microcystic lesion with honeycomb appearance
  - Treatment: Observation unless symptomatic

Mucinous cystic neoplasms (MCN):

- More commonly found in the body or tail of the pancreas
  - Mucinous cystadenoma—benign
  - Mucinous cystadenocarcinoma—malignant
  - Treatment: Resection. Even for benign mucinous cystic neoplasms, treatment is resection since there is potential for malignant transformation

Intraductal mucinous papillary neoplasm (IPMN):

- More commonly found in the head of pancreas with duct involvement
  - May visualize mucin coming from the ampulla
  - Treatment: Resection. May be multifocal in nature, perform frozen section intraoperatively to ensure margins are negative

RADIOLOGY

Hypodense Lesion at the Tail of the Pancreas

- **Plain film findings**
  - Usually normal
- **CT findings** (Fig. 6.4)
  - Pancreatic tumor protocol includes nonenhanced, late arterial, and portal venous phases
  - For pancreatic adenocarcinomas, arterial phase images demonstrate a hypodense pancreatic lesion with respect to the normal pancreas

  For pancreatic islet cell tumors, arterial phase images demonstrate a hyperenhancing mass with respect to the normal pancreas

  portal venous phase images can help to detect extent of disease in the abdomen (i.e. metastatic disease, local invasion)

FIGURE 6.4 A–C

A. Liver
B. Kidney
C. Vertebra
D. Small bowel loops
E. Gallbladder
F. Descending aorta
G. Spleen
H. Portal vein
I. Stomach
J. Renal artery

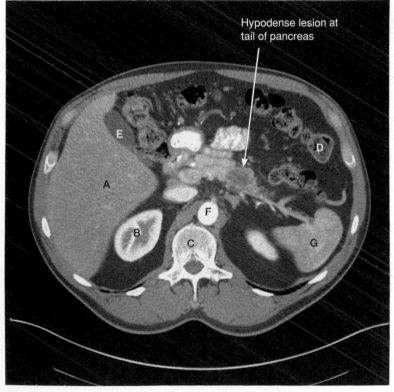

Hypodense lesion at tail of pancreas

FIGURE 6.4 A

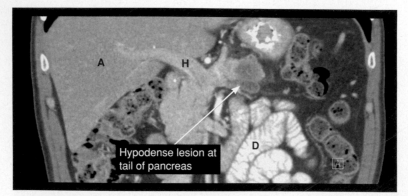

FIGURE 6.4 B

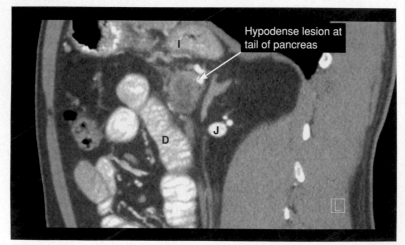

FIGURE 6.4 C

Pancreatic Tumor at the Head of the Pancreas

- **Plain film findings**
  - If the mass is large, there may be widening of the duodenal loop, irregularity of the inner border
- **US findings**
  - Hypoechoic mass within the pancreatic head
  - May be associated with pancreatic and/or biliary duct dilation
- **CT findings** (Fig. 6.5)
  - Hypoenhancing mass, lower in density than the normal pancreas
  - Islet cell tumors are typically hyperenhancing with respect to the pancreas
  - May be associated with biliary or pancreatic ductal dilatation (double-duct sign)
- **MRI findings**
  - Adenocarcinomas are usually hypoenhancing with respect to the normal pancreas on contrast T1-weighted images
  - Islet cell tumors are usually hyperenhancing with respect to the normal pancreas on contrast T1-weighted images
  - Usually T2 hyperintense

FIGURE 6.5 A–C

A. Liver

B. Gallbladder

C. Descending aorta

D. Kidney

E. Vertebra

F. Spleen

G. Small bowel loops

H. Stomach

I. Portal vein

J. Body of pancreas

K. IVC

L. Common bile duct

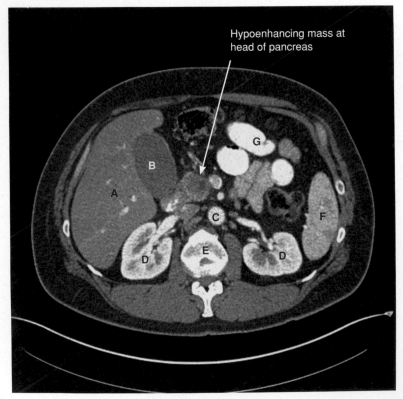

Hypoenhancing mass at head of pancreas

FIGURE 6.5 A

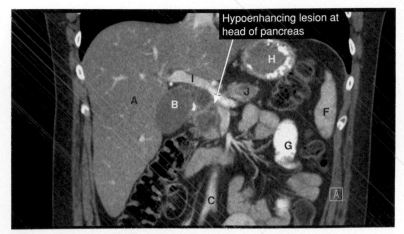

FIGURE 6.5 B

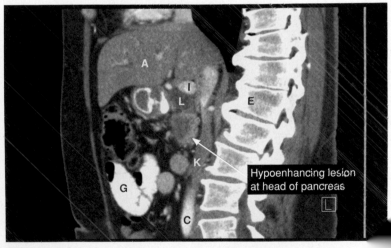

FIGURE 6.5 C

Invasive Pancreatic Tumor

- **CT findings** (Fig. 6.6)
  - Hypoenhancing mass in the head of pancreas with soft tissue surrounding structures such as superior mesenteric artery, bile duct, etc.

FIGURE 6.6 A–C

A. Liver   E. Small bowel loops

B. IVC   F. Stomach

C. Vertebra   G. Body of pancreas

D. Kidney   H. Portal vein

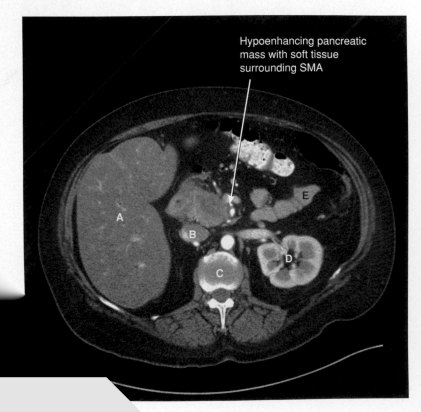

Hypoenhancing pancreatic mass with soft tissue surrounding SMA

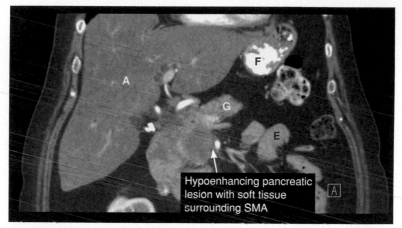

Hypoenhancing pancreatic lesion with soft tissue surrounding SMA

FIGURE 6.6 B

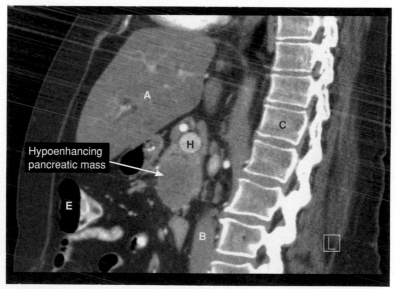

Hypoenhancing pancreatic mass

FIGURE 6.6 C

Suggested Readings

Aghdassi A, Mayerle J, Kraft M, et al. Diagnosis and treatment of pancreatic pseudocysts in chronic pancreatitis. *Pancreas.* 2008;36(2):105–112.

Balthazar EJ. Acute pancreatitis: Assessment of severity with clinical and CT evaluation. *Radiology.* 2002;223:603–613.

Brennan DD, Zamboni GA, Raptopoulos VD, et al. Comprehensive preoperative assessment of pancreatic adenocarcinoma with 64-section volumetric CT. *Radiographics.* 2007;27:1653–1666.

Callery MP, Chang KJ, Fishman EK, et al. Pretreatment assessment of resectable and borderline resectable pancreatic cancer: Expert consensus statement. *Ann Surg Oncol.* 2009;16(7):1727–1733.

Habashi S, Draganov PV. Pancreatic pseudocyst. *World J Gastroenterol.* 2009;15(1): 38–47.

Kim YH, Saini S, Sahani D, et al. Imaging diagnosis of cystic pancreatic lesions: Pseudocyst versus nonpseudocyst. *Radiographics.* 2005;25:671–685.

Mortele KJ, Girshman J, Szejnfeld D, et al. CT-guided percutaneous catheter drainage of acute necrotizing pancreatitis: Clinical experience and observations in patients with sterile and infected necrosis. *AJR Am J Roentgenol.* 2009;192:110–116.

Tamm EP, Silverman PM, Charnsangavej C, et al. Diagnosis, staging, and surveillance of pancreatic cancer. *AJR Am J Roentgenol.* 2003;180:1311–1323.

Tonsi AF, Bacchion M, Crippa S, et al. Acute pancreatitis at the beginning of the 21st century: The state of the art. *World J Gastroenterol.* 2009;15(24):2945–2959.

Villatoro E, Mulla M, Larvin M. Antibiotic therapy for prophylaxis against infection of pancreatic necrosis in acute pancreatitis. *Cochrane Database Syst Rev.* 2010;(5):CD002941.

7

Small Bowel

Small Bowel Obstruction

Overview

- Most commonly due to adhesions (70%) or incarceration of bowel within a hernia
- Other etiologies include small bowel tumor, volvulus, intussusception, and strictures
- Obstruction may be partial or complete

Signs and Symptoms

- Colicky periumbilical pain that may be relieved with bilious emesis
- Abdominal distention, tenderness, and occasional high-pitched bowel sounds
- Severe tenderness at the site of incarcerated hernia with possible overlying skin changes
- Patients with complete bowel obstruction will have absence of flatus or bowel movement, patients with partial bowel obstruction will present with abdominal distention with decreased passage of flatus

Diagnosis

- Abdominal x-rays will show multiple air–fluid levels with diste͏ loops of small bowel
- CT scan with IV contrast may be obtained to assess for a t͏ point

Treatment/Management

■ NPO for bowel rest, IV fluids, NG decompression; correct any underlying electrolyte abnormalities

■ Attempt to perform bedside reduction of any incarcerated hernia

■ Patients with diffuse peritonitis or complete bowel obstruction should warrant surgical exploration

■ Patients with partial bowel obstruction who do not improve with conservative management will require exploration and adhesiolysis with possible bowel resection

■ Patients without signs of incarcerated hernia and who have no previous abdominal surgeries should also be surgically explored

RADIOLOGY

■ **Plain film findings** (Fig. 7.1)

• Dilated small bowel loops with air fluid levels

■ **CT findings** (Fig. 7.1)

• Fluid-filled, dilated small bowel loops

• Closed-loop obstruction manifests as a C-shaped configuration of dilated bowel loops with mesenteric vessels converging toward the point of torsion

• Strangulation is characterized by bowel wall thickening, little or no contrast enhancement of the bowel wall, engorgement of mesenteric vasculature, and mesenteric edema

• Small bowel loops are dilated proximal to the obstruction, and decompressed distal to the obstruction

FIGURE 7.1 A–H

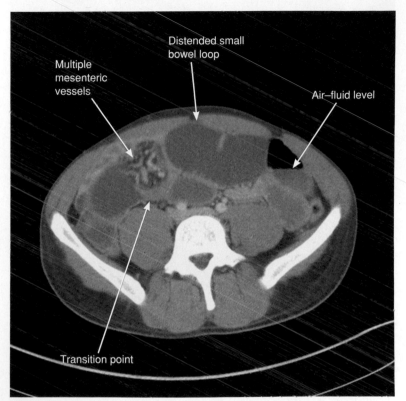

FIGURE 7.1 A

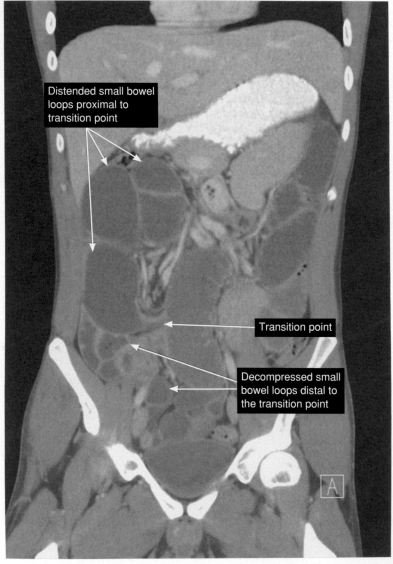

Distended small bowel loops proximal to transition point

Transition point

Decompressed small bowel loops distal to the transition point

FIGURE 7.1 B

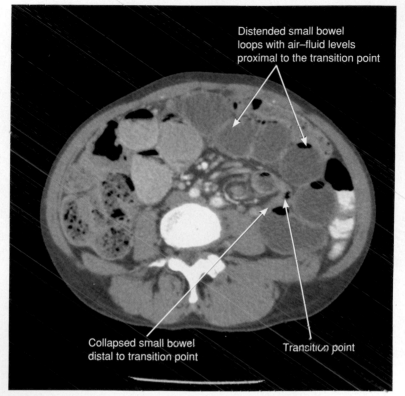

Distended small bowel loops with air–fluid levels proximal to the transition point

Collapsed small bowel distal to transition point

Transition point

FIGURE 7.1 C

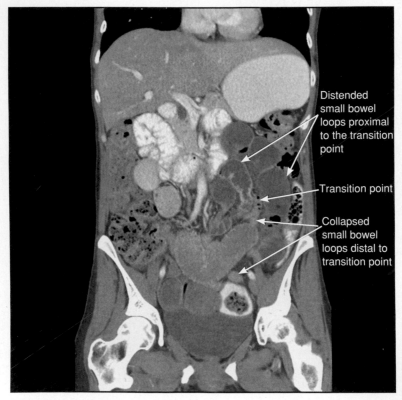

Distended small bowel loops proximal to the transition point

Transition point

Collapsed small bowel loops distal to transition point

FIGURE 7.1 D

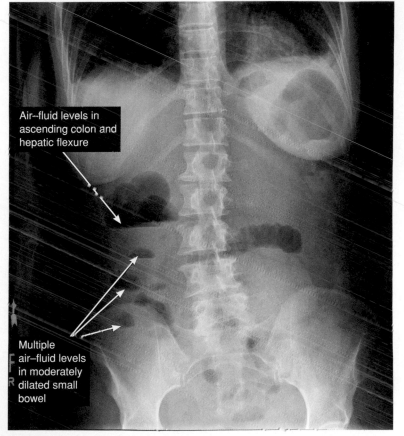

Air–fluid levels in ascending colon and hepatic flexure

Multiple air–fluid levels in moderately dilated small bowel

FIGURE 7.1 E

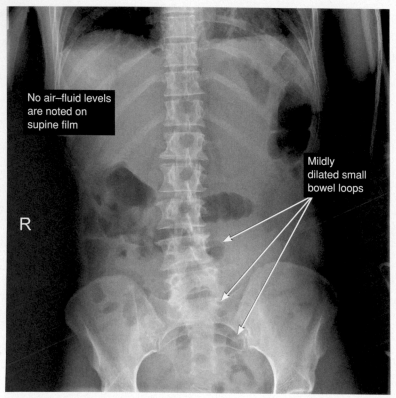

No air–fluid levels are noted on supine film

Mildly dilated small bowel loops

R

FIGURE 7.1 F

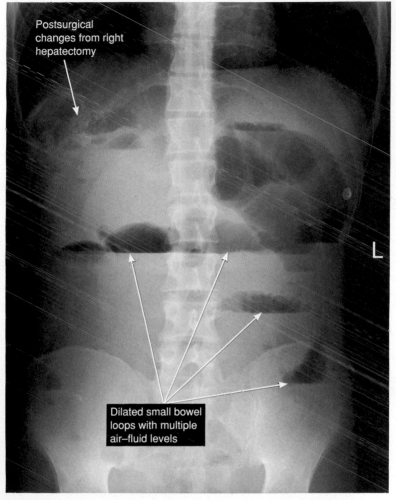

Postsurgical changes from right hepatectomy

L

Dilated small bowel loops with multiple air–fluid levels

FIGURE 7.1 G

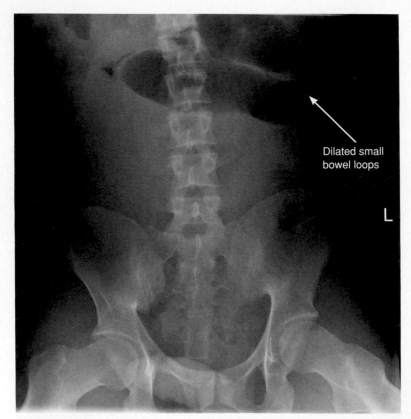

FIGURE 7.1 H

Ileus

Overview

- Lack of peristalsis or bowel function without a structural obstruction
- Most commonly secondary to abdominal surgery
- Other causes are electrolyte abnormalities, intra-abdominal abscess, systemic infection, hypothyroidism, or other medications such as anticholinergics

Signs and Symptoms

- Abdominal distension without flatus or bowel movements
- Bilious or feculent emesis
- Generalized abdominal distension associated with discomfort without diffuse peritonitis

Diagnosis

- Same as small bowel obstruction

Treatment/Management

- Same as small bowel obstruction
- May consider initiation of total parenteral nutrition (TPN) for patients who have prolonged ileus with underlying malnutrition

RADIOLOGY

- **Plain film findings** (Fig. 7.2)
  - Distended small bowel loops with air fluid levels
  - May be indistinguishable from SBO
  - Distal air in the rectum may help differentiate ileus from SBO

FIGURE 7.2 A,B
_____

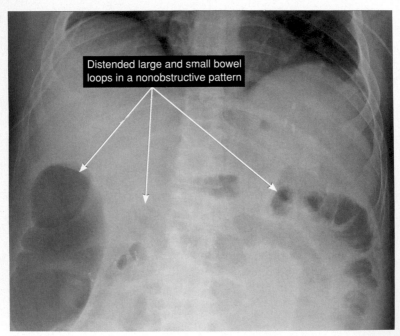

Distended large and small bowel loops in a nonobstructive pattern

FIGURE 7.2 A

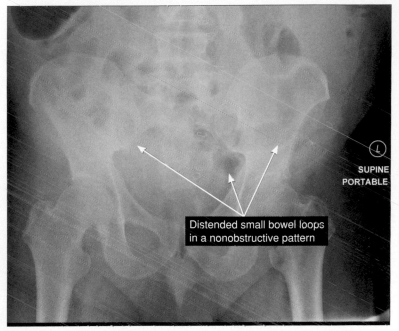

FIGURE 7.2 B

Small Bowel Enterocutaneous Fistula

Overview

- A fistula is defined as an abnormal connection between two epithelized organs
- Small bowel enterocutaneous fistula is usually caused by unrecognized iatrogenic injury to the bowel, anastomotic leak, inflammatory bowel disease, or malignancy

Signs and Symptoms

- Fever, leukocytosis, ileus, abdominal tenderness followed by drainage of enteric contents via the wound or skin
- Factors that prevent fistula closure—(FRIEND)
  - **F**oreign body
  - **R**adiation
  - **I**nflammation/infection
  - **E**pithelialization of the tract
  - **N**eoplasm
  - **D**istal obstruction

Diagnosis

- CT scan with enteric contrast will help identify any undrained abscess. It might help identify the origin of the fistula
- Fistulogram or sinogram consists of contrast injection into the cutaneous end of the fistula to evaluate the tract and origin of the fistula

Treatment/Management

- Usually treatment consists of making patient NPO, parenteral nutrition, possible octreotide to decrease the output from the fistula for easier wound management
- Definitive treatment is surgery if spontaneous closure does not occur within 4 to 5 weeks' time

RADIOLOGY

- **Plain film findings**
  - Contrast injection through the fistula can diagnose the tract between the skin and the small bowel lumen
- **CT findings** (Fig. 7.3)
  - CT can be performed in addition to a fistulogram to distinguish fluid collections from bowel loops, and also to guide percutaneous drainage of any abscesses
    - A fistula between the small bowel and skin can sometimes be directly seen on CT
    - stranding and abscess formation may be seen around the tract

FIGURE 7.3 A–C

A. Stomach
B. Descending colon
C. Portal vein
D. Liver
E. Mesenteric vessels
F. Psoas muscle

G. IVC
H. Common iliac artery
I. Small bowel loops
J. Vertebra
K. Kidney

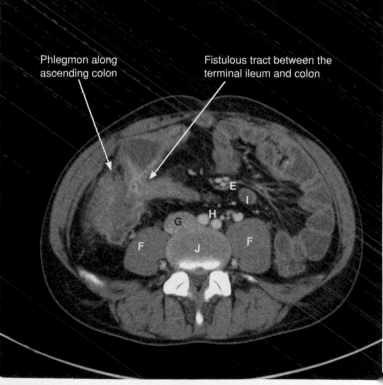

Phlegmon along ascending colon

Fistulous tract between the terminal ileum and colon

FIGURE 7.3 A

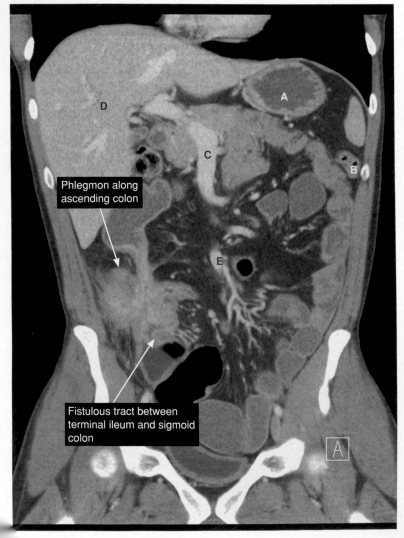

Phlegmon along ascending colon

Fistulous tract between terminal ileum and sigmoid colon

FIGURE 7.3 B

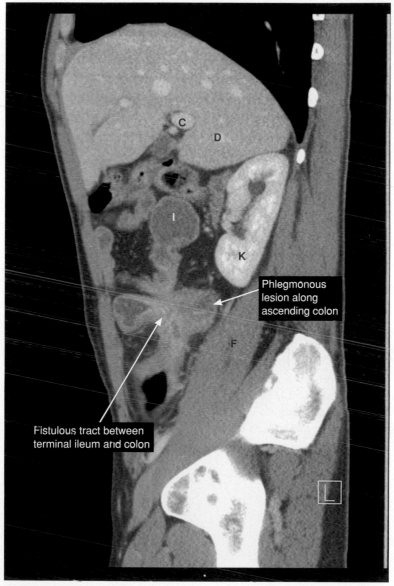

Phlegmonous
lesion along
ascending colon

Fistulous tract between
terminal ileum and colon

FIGURE 7.3 C

Pneumatosis Intestinalis

Overview

- Presence of gas within the wall of the intestine
- Usually a sign of acute mesenteric ischemia
- May be idiopathic in nature, especially in a stable patient without abdominal pain or signs of sepsis

Diagnosis

- CT scan shows air within the bowel wall

Treatment/Management

- Mesenteric ischemia: Resect nonviable bowel
- Idiopathic: Observation, serial abdominal examination, possible surgical exploration if patient decompensates

---

KEY POINTS

- This is a radiologic finding that may be seen even on plain films. May also be associated with free air or portal venous gas
- The progression of air within the walls should be of concern. In questionable cases, diagnostic laparoscopy may act as a mode of surgical exploration without the morbidity of a negative exploratory laparotomy

RADIOLOGY

- **Plain film findings** (Fig. 7.4)
  - Pneumatosis appears as bubbly or linear lucencies in the bowel wall associated with dilated bowel loops
  - Portal venous gas in the liver may be seen in minority of cases
  - Resolution of intramural or portal venous gas may indicate perforation rather than recovery
- **CT findings** (Fig. 7.5)
  - Linear or bubbly gas within the bowel wall
  - Intraluminal bowel contents mixed with air can mimic pneumatosis intestinalis
  - Viewing the bowel loops in lung windows is useful for identifying gas within the bowel wall
  - May be associated with bowel wall thickening, mesenteric vessel occlusion, dilated bowel, ascites, portomesenteric venous gas
  - Pneumatosis confined to a short segment of bowel suggests vascular occlusion as the etiology

Pneumatosis Intestinalis in a Pediatric

FIGURE 7.4 A,B

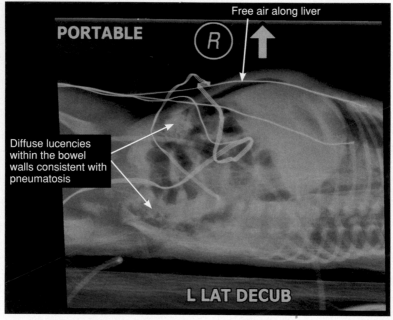

FIGURE 7.4 A

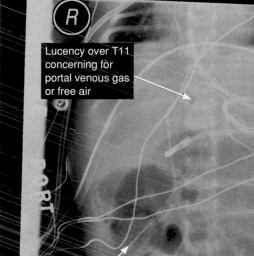

Lucency over T11 concerning for portal venous gas or free air

Pneumatosis at splenic flexure

Pneumatosis involving right side of abdomen

AP
PORTABLE
SUPINE

FIGURE 7.4 B

Pneumatosis Intestinalis

FIGURE 7.5 A–C

A. Vertebra	E. Liver
B. Descending aorta	F. Stomach
C. IVC	G. Spleen
D. Small bowel loops	H. Ascites

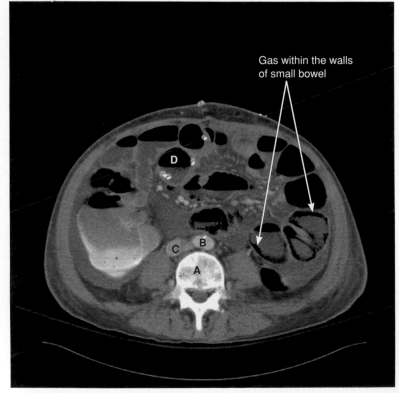

Gas within the walls of small bowel

FIGURE 7.5 A

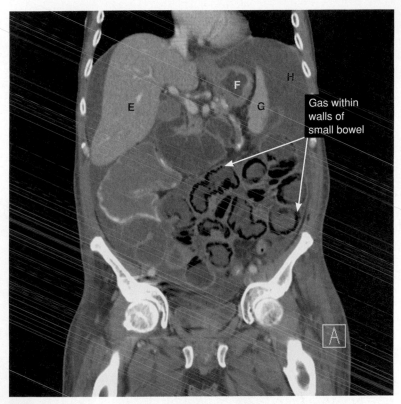

Gas within walls of small bowel

FIGURE 7.5 B

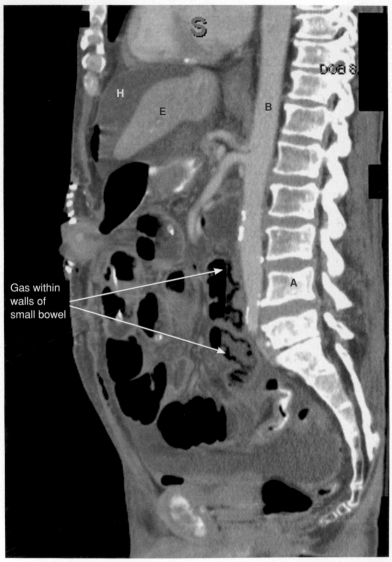

Gas within walls of small bowel

FIGURE 7.5 C

Meckel's Diverticulum

Overview

- Remnant of the omphalomesenteric duct (vitelline duct)
- True diverticulum involving all layers of the bowel, found on the antimesenteric side of the bowel
- Rule of 2's: 2% of the population, 2 feet from the ileocecal valve, 2 inches in length, most commonly at 2 years of age, 2:1 male to female ratio, 2 types of ectopic tissue (gastric and pancreatic)

Signs and Symptoms

- Most common presentation in pediatric population is painless bleeding
- Most common presentation in adults is abdominal pain due to intestinal obstruction

Diagnosis

- Meckel scan (technetium-99m pertechnetate scan) is sensitive in detecting ectopic gastric tissue. Ideal for pediatric patients, less accurate in adults
- Small bowel follow through and enteroclysis are 75% accurate
- Most of the time, it is discovered incidentally on a CT scan or during surgery

Treatment/Management

- Segmental ileal resection
- For asymptomatic or incidental diverticulum, it is controversial whether segmental bowel resection or diverticulectomy should be performed

RADIOLOGY

- **Plain film findings**
  - Usually normal
- **CT findings** (Fig. 7.6)
  - Tubular fluid containing structure communicating with the small bowel
  - Fat stranding around the diverticulum may be present

FIGURE 7.6 A,B

A. Psoas muscle	E. Liver
B. Small bowel loops	F. Gallbladder
C. Large bowel	G. Stomach
D. Vertebra	

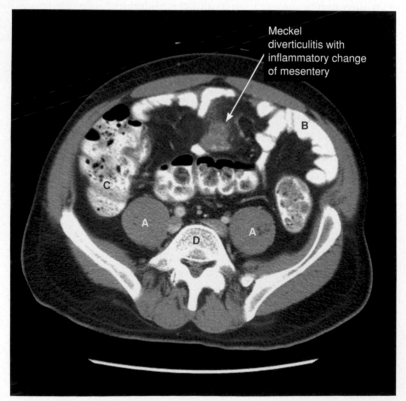

Meckel diverticulitis with inflammatory change of mesentery

FIGURE 7.6 A

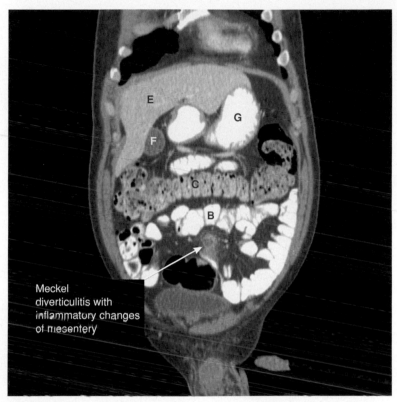

Meckel diverticulitis with inflammatory changes of mesentery

FIGURE 7.6 B

Intussusception

Overview

- Telescoping or invagination of one segment of intestine into another
- In the pediatric population, it is one of the frequent causes of bowel obstruction
  - Most are idiopathic intussusceptions. If lead point is present, it is rarely pathologic in nature, such as a Meckel diverticulum or hypertrophic Peyer patches in the terminal ileum
- In the adult population, intussusception is mostly associated with a pathologic lead point such as a tumor or polyp

Signs and Symptoms

- Children present with "redcurrant jelly" stool and palpable sausage-shaped abdominal mass
- Adults present with signs and symptoms similar to bowel obstruction

Diagnosis

- Abdominal ultrasound
- CT scan demonstrates a "target sign"

Treatment/Management

- **For pediatric patients**
  - Intussusception may be reduced by air or contrast enema
  - If unsuccessful, then surgery for manual reduction and resection of lead point if present
- **For adults**
  - Conservative treatment for those who present with incidental radiologic findings of intussusception
  - For those with worsening abdominal pain, signs of bowel obstruction or mass noted on imaging, surgical exploration is warranted

RADIOLOGY

- **Plain film findings**
  - Submucosal masses such as an underlying malignancy can precipitate an intussusception
  - A soft tissue mass outlined by gas may be seen

- **CT findings** (Fig. 7.7)
  - Diagnosed by the intussusceptum bringing mesenteric fat through the lumen of the intussuscipiens
  - Can appear as a sausage-shaped or targetoid mass
  - Underlying cause for the intussusception may also be apparent (such as a lipoma)
  - In ileocolic intussusceptions, the ileocecal valve protrudes into the cecum

FIGURE 7.7 A–C

A. Psoas muscle D. Air within small bowel
B. Vertebra   E. Liver
C. Small bowel loops F. Kidney

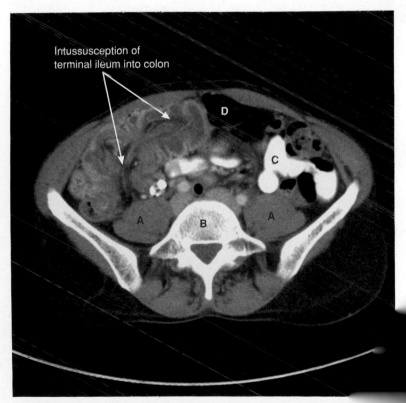

FIGURE 7.7 A

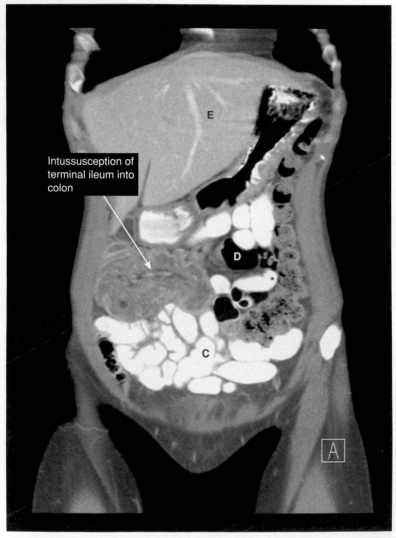

Intussusception of terminal ileum into colon

FIGURE 7.7 B

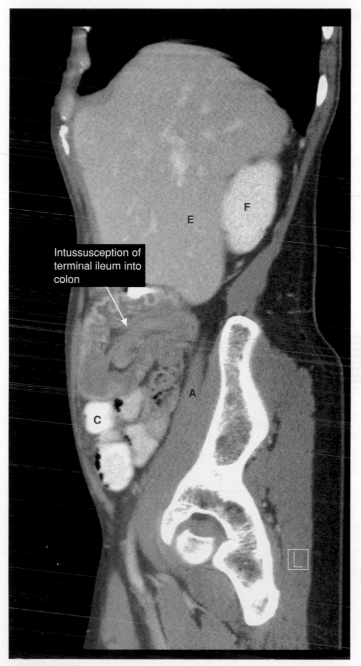

Intussusception of terminal ileum into colon

FIGURE 7.7 C

Mesenteric Ischemia

Overview

- Etiologies include: embolic, acute thrombosis, chronic mesenteric ischemia, venous thrombosis, nonocclusive or low flow state, and iatrogenic injury
- Most common etiology: Embolic

Signs and Symptoms

- Abdominal pain out of proportion to physical examination findings, nausea, vomiting, abdominal distension, bloody stools
- Leukocytosis with left shift, lactic acidosis (may be a late manifestation)

Diagnosis

- Mostly a clinical diagnosis
- If there is a high clinical suspicion, imaging would be helpful

Treatment/Management

- OR for embolectomy and possible bowel resection

KEY POINT
- Angiography is the gold standard, but CT angiography is the most convenient

---

RADIOLOGY

- **Plain film findings**
  - May see ileus secondary to ischemia

- **CT findings** (Fig. 7.8)
  - Vessel thrombus manifests as intraluminal filling defect
  - Bowel distention and bowel wall thickening are often seen
  - Submucosal edema will appear as hypoattenuation within the bowel wall
  - Ascites may be present
  - Pneumatosis usually suggests necrotic bowel

FIGURE 7.8 A–C

A. Abdominal ascites   E. Small bowel loops
B. Liver   F. Descending aorta
C. Kidneys   G. Gallbladder
D. Vertebra

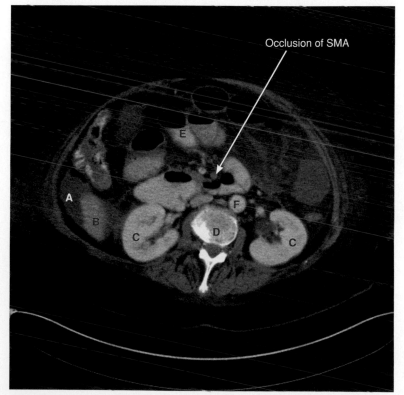

FIGURE 7.8 A

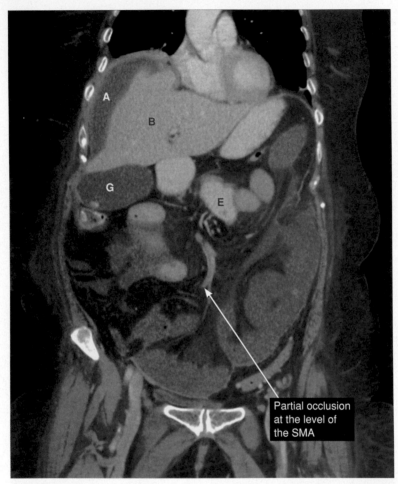

Partial occlusion at the level of the SMA

FIGURE 7.8 B

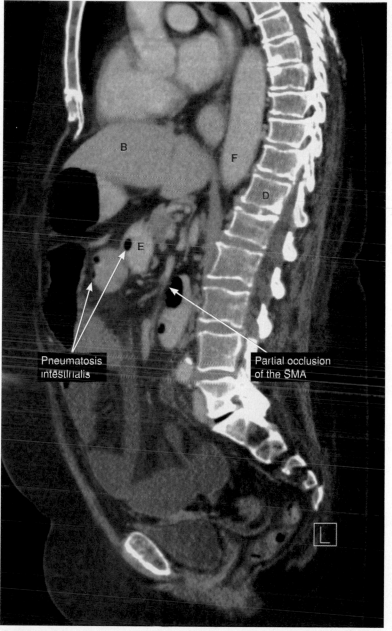

FIGURE 7.8 C

Suggested Readings

Azar T, Berger DL. Adult intussusception. *Ann Surg.* 1997;226(2):134–138.

Demirkan A, Yagmurlu A, Kepenekci I, et al. Intussusception in adult and pediatric patients: Two different entities. *Surg Today.* 2009;39(10):861–865.

Eisen LK, Cunningham JD, Aufses AH Jr. Intussusception in adults: Institutional review. *J Am Coll Surg.* 1999;188(4):390–395.

Evenson AR, Fischer JE. Current management of enterocutaneous fistula. *J Gastrointest Surg.* 2006;10(3):455–464.

Frager DH, Baer JW, Rothpearl A, et al. Distinction between postoperative ileus and mechanical small-bowel obstruction: Value of CT compared with clinical and other radiographic findings. *AJR Am J Roentgenol.* 1995;164:891–894.

Furukawa A, Kanasaki S, Kono N, et al. CT diagnosis of acute mesenteric ischemia from various causes. *AJR Am J Roentgenol.* 2009;192:408–416.

Gayer G, Zissin R, Apter S, et al. Pictorial review: Adult intussusception–a CT diagnosis. *Br J Radiol.* 2002;75:185–190.

Ho LM, Paulson EK, Thompson WM. Pneumatosis intestinalis in the adult: Benign to life-threatening causes. *AJR Am J Roentgenol.* 2007;188:1604–1613.

Kaiser AD, Applegate KE, Ladd AP. Current success in the treatment of intussusception in children. *Surgery.* 2007;142(4):469–475.

Laine L, Jensen DM. Management of patients with ulcer bleeding. *Am J Gastroenterol.* 2012;107(3):345–360.

Lunevicius R, Morkevicius M. Comparison of laparoscopic versus open repair for perforated duodenal ulcers. *Surg Endosc.* 2005;19(12):1565–1571.

Oldenburg WA, Lau LL, Rodenberg TJ, et al. Acute mesenteric ischemia: A clinical review. *Arch Intern Med.* 2004;164(10):1054–1062.

Park JJ, Wolff BG, Tollefson MK, et al. Meckel diverticulum: The Mayo Clinic experience with 1476 patients (1950–2002). *Ann Surg.* 2005;241(3):529–533.

Paulsen SR, Huprich JE, Fletcher JG, et al. CT enterography as a diagnostic tool in evaluating small bowel disorders: Review of clinical experience with over 700 cases. *Radiographics.* 2006;26:641–657.

Pickhardt PJ, Bhalla S, Balfe DM. Acquired gastrointestinal fistulas: Classification, etiologies, and imaging evaluation. *Radiology.* 2002;224:9–23.

Rea JD, Lockhart ME, Yarbrough DE, et.al. Approach to management of intussusception in adults: A new paradigm in the computed tomography era. *Am Surg.* 2007;73(11):1098–1105.

Renner P, Kienle K, Dahlke MH, et al. Intestinal ischemia: Current treatment concepts. *Langenbecks Arch Surg.* 2011;396(1):3–11.

Ruscher KA, Fisher JN, Hughes CD, et al. National trends in the surgical management of Meckel's diverticulum. *J Pediatr Surg.* 2011;46(5):893–896.

Satya R, O'Malley JP. Case 86: Meckel diverticulum with massive bleeding. *Radiology.* 2005;236:836–840.

Wayne E, Ough M, Wu A, et al. Management algorithm for pneumatosis intestinalis and portal venous gas: Treatment and outcome of 88 consecutive cases. *J Gastrointest Surg.* 2010;14(3):437–448.

Williams LJ, Zolfaghari S, Boushey RP. Complications of enterocutaneous fistulas and their management. *Clin Colon Rectal Surg.* 2010;23(3):209–220.

Zissin R, Osadchy A, Gayer G, et al. Pictorial review. CT of duodenal pathology. *Br J Radiol.* 2002;75:78–84.

8

Large Bowel

Diverticular Diseases

Overview

- Diverticula are outpouchings of the mucosa through the colonic wall. Usually located at the area of colonic wall that is traversed by arterioles (vasa recta)
- False diverticulum includes only mucosa and submucosa
- May lead to perforation or bleeding

Signs and Symptoms

- Abdominal pain, fever, leukocytosis, lower GI bleeding

Diagnosis

- Hinchey classification of perforated diverticular disease:
  - Class I: Perforation with localized paracolonic abscess
  - Class II: Perforation with pelvic abscess
  - Class III: Perforation with purulent peritonitis
  - Class IV: Perforation with feculent peritonitis
- Diverticulitis: CT scan with IV contrast. Water-soluble rectal contrast is relatively contraindicated in the setting of acute diverticulitis
- Lower GI bleed from diverticula: Colonoscopy, visceral angiography, tagged red blood cell scan

Treatment/Management

- Diverticulitis with no diffuse peritonitis: Conservative treatment with bowel rest, antibiotics
- Recurrent diverticulitis: Cut off for timing of surgery still a controversial debate, but most patients are offered resection if they have had more than three episodes of diverticulitis;failure to resolve an episode despite medical management; complicated diverticulitis (for example: perforation with abscess formation, colovesicular fistula, etc); or if the attacks are increasing in severity or frequency
- Abscess: IR drainage
- Bleeding: Resuscitation, therapeutic colonoscopy, IR embolization, surgical resection for persistent, or the rare case of uncontrollable bleeding

RADIOLOGY

Diverticulosis

- **CT findings** (Fig. 8.1)
  - Focal outpouchings from the colonic wall without surrounding inflammation (which would indicate diverticulitis)

FIGURE 8.1 A–E

A. Psoas muscle
B. Vertebra
C. Small bowel loops
D. Liver

E. Stomach
F. Spleen
G. Descending aorta
H. Bladder

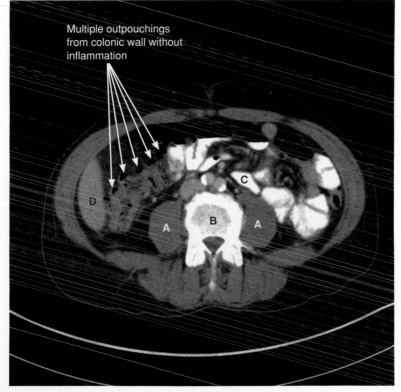

Multiple outpouchings from colonic wall without inflammation

FIGURE 8.1 A

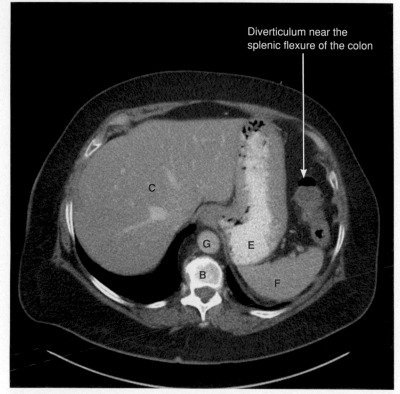

Diverticulum near the splenic flexure of the colon

FIGURE 8.1 B

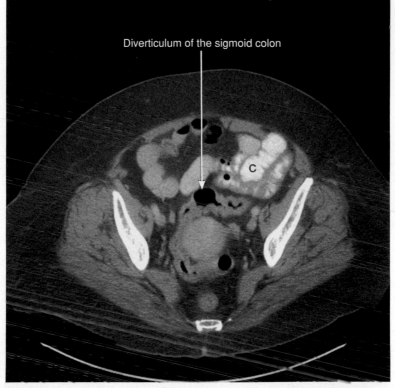

Diverticulum of the sigmoid colon

C

FIGURE 8.1 C

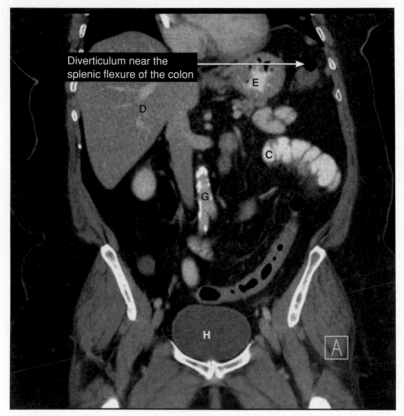

FIGURE 8.1 D

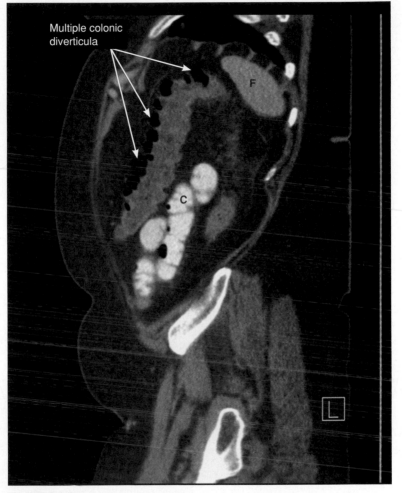

FIGURE 8.1 E

Diverticulitis

- **Plain film findings**
  - Usually normal, but may see thickened loops of colon
- **US findings**
  - May reveal a pericolic abscess as a hypoechoic fluid collection with posterior acoustic enhancement near the bowel wall, surrounded by inflamed hyperechoic fat
- **CT findings** (Fig. 8.2)
  - Pericolonic fat stranding and edema
  - May see a loculated, rim enhancing fluid collection, representing an abscess
  - Colonic wall thickening secondary to inflammation
  - Mild disease is characterized by minimal wall thickening and pericolonic inflammatory changes
  - Moderate disease is characterized by the formation of pericolonic fluid collections, representing abscesses
  - Severe disease is characterized by marked wall thickening, large amount of free air, large fluid collections, or marked phlegmonous changes

FIGURE 8.2 A,B

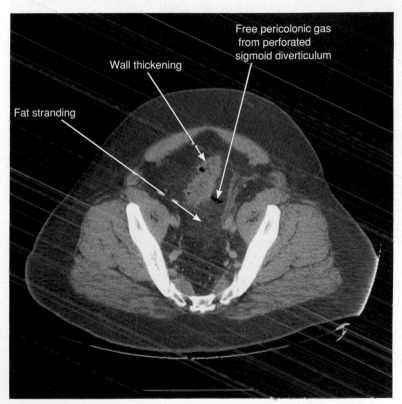

FIGURE 8.2 A

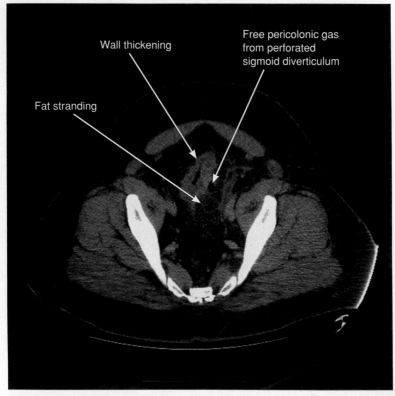

FIGURE 8.2 B

Perforated Diverticulitis

- **CT findings** (Fig. 8.3)
  - Free intraperitoneal air
  - Pericolonic fat stranding surrounding the perforated diverticuli

---

FIGURE 8.3 A–D

A. Psoas muscle
B. Vertebra
C. Small bowel loops
D. Liver

E. Stomach
F. Bladder
G. Kidney

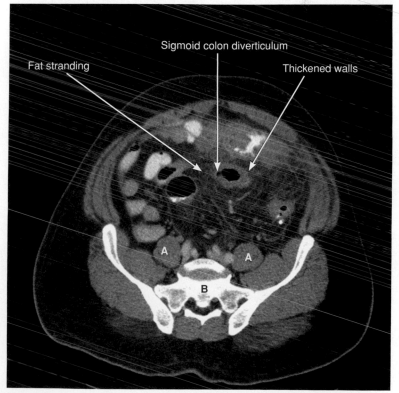

FIGURE 8.3 A

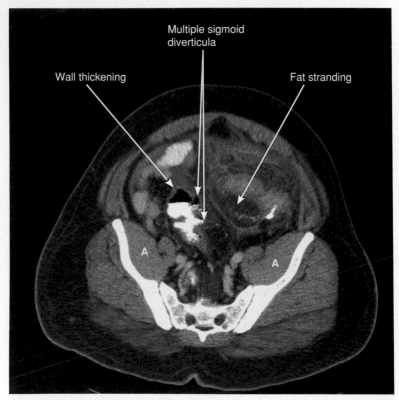

FIGURE 8.3 B

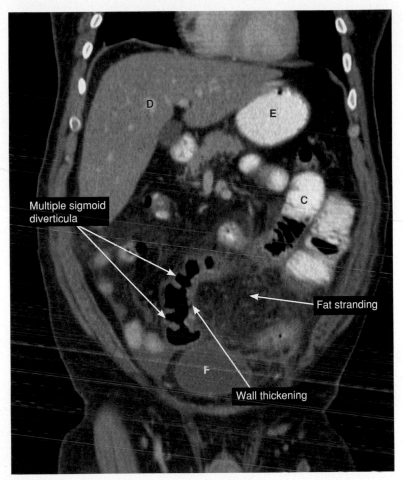

FIGURE 8.3 C

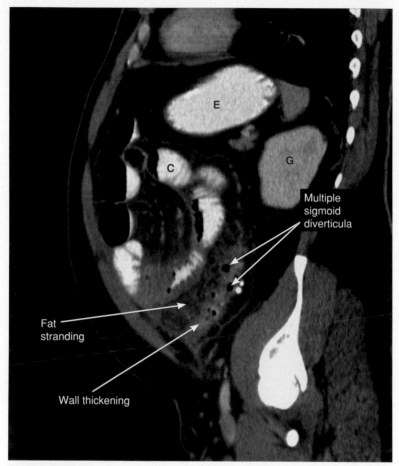

FIGURE 8.3 D

Diverticular Pelvic Abscess

- **CT findings** (Fig. 8.4)
  - Loculated, rim-enhancing fluid collection around the site of diverticulitis
  - Extensive surrounding fat stranding

FIGURE 8.4 A–C

A. Sacrum	G. Descending aorta
B. Ilium	H. IVC
C. Fat stranding	I. Portal vein
D. Liver	J. Vertebra
E. Small bowel loops	K. Uterus
F. Bladder	

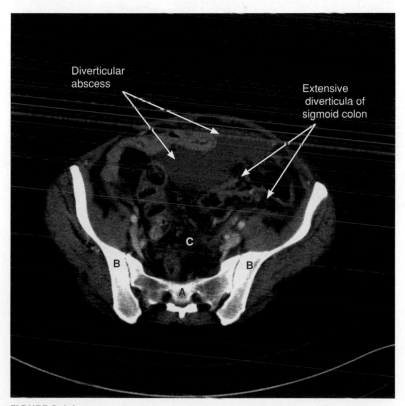

FIGURE 8.4 A

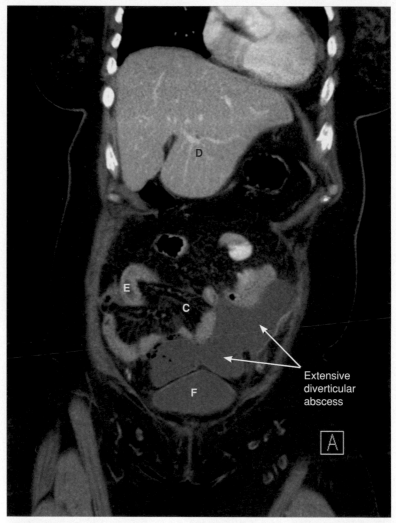

Extensive diverticular abscess

FIGURE 8.4 B

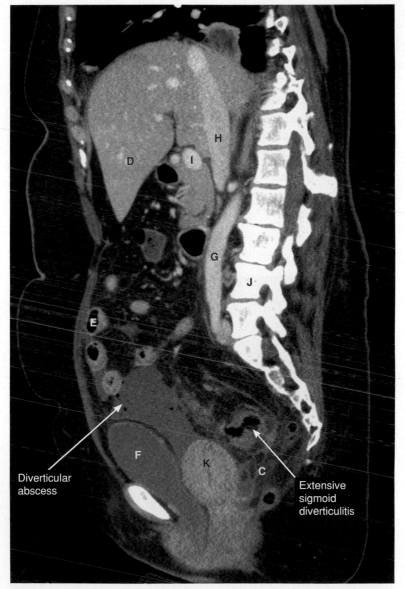

Diverticular abscess

Extensive sigmoid diverticulitis

FIGURE 8.4 C

Colovesicular Fistula

RADIOLOGY

- **CT findings** (Fig. 8.5)
  - Gas within the bladder
  - Focal wall thickening of the bladder
  - Tethering of the colon to the bladder is usually seen. The fistula tract is usually not seen on CT

FIGURE 8.5 A–C

A. Rectum
B. Femoral head
C. Liver
D. Stomach
E. Small bowel loops

F. Urinary bladder
G. Superior mesenteric vein
H. Descending aorta
I. Vertebra

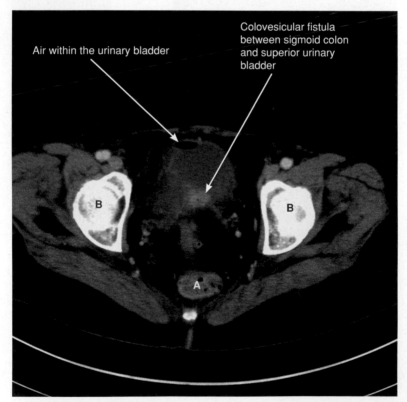

Air within the urinary bladder

Colovesicular fistula between sigmoid colon and superior urinary bladder

FIGURE 8.5 A

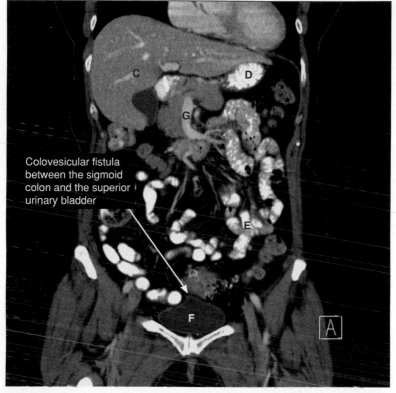

Colovesicular fistula
between the sigmoid
colon and the superior
urinary bladder

FIGURE 8.5 B

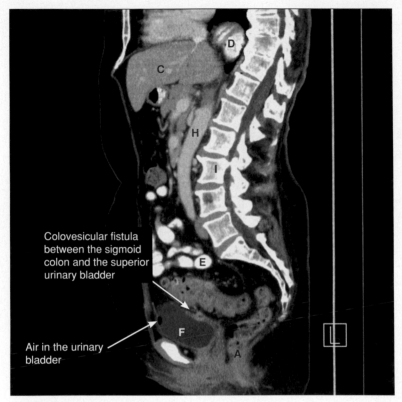

Colovesicular fistula between the sigmoid colon and the superior urinary bladder

Air in the urinary bladder

FIGURE 8.5 C

Colorectal Cancer

- **Hereditary colorectal cancer syndromes**
  - Make up 5% to 10% of all colorectal cancers
  - Autosomal dominant
- **Hereditary nonpolyposis colorectal cancer (HNPCC) also known as Lynch syndrome**
  - Most common inherited colorectal cancer (2% to 4% colorectal cancers)
  - Amsterdam criteria
    - Three relatives with histologically proven colorectal CA (one first degree)
    - Two successive generations
    - One diagnosed prior to the age of 50 years

- DNA mismatch repair
- 50% to 85% lifetime risk of colon cancer
- Extracolonic manifestation: Tumors of endometrium, ovaries, stomach, small bowel, hepatobiliary tract, pancreas, ureter, renal pelvis

- **Familial adenomatous polyposis (FAP)**
  - Second most common familial colorectal cancer
  - Hundreds to thousands of adenomatous polyps
  - APC gene mutation chromosome 5
  - Almost all patients will develop colon cancer
  - Mean age polyposis at 15 years of age
  - Extracolonic manifestation: Duodenal polyps (periampullary cancer), desmoid tumors, epidermoid cyst, mandibular osteomas (Gardner's syndrome), central nervous system tumors (Turcot syndrome)

- **Attenuated FAP**
  - Fewer polyps
  - Later age onset (30 years)
  - 70% lifetime risk for colon cancer

- **Peutz–Jeghers syndrome**
  - Hamartomatous polyps
  - Polyps of small intestine, rectum, colon
  - Melanin spots in buccal surface

- **Juvenile polyposis syndrome**
  - Hamartomatous polyps
  - Hundreds of polyps in rectum or colon
  - May degenerate into adenoma and carcinoma

Diagnosis

- Screening
  - For average risk start screening at the age of 50 years
  - More frequent screening if history of polyps, colon cancer, inflammatory bowel disease, family history of colon cancer
- Preoperative evaluation
  - CT chest, abdomen, pelvis
  - Colonoscopy (synchronous tumors ~5%)

- Rectal cancer—endorectal ultrasound
- CEA level

Treatment/Management

- Resection
- Twelve lymph nodes required for adequate staging
- ± adjuvant chemotherapy

RADIOLOGY

Colon Cancer

- **Plain film/contrast enema findings**
  - Annular cancers manifest as shouldering with an irregular narrow lumen
  - Polypoid cancers usually present as intraluminal masses that protrude from the wall into the lumen of the colon
  - Obstruction is much more common on the left due to its smaller caliber compared to the right hemicolon
- **CT findings** (Fig. 8.6)
  - Enhancement of cancer
  - Heterogeneous enhancement with abscess formation (secondary to perforation)
  - Calcification may be seen with mucinous adenocarcinomas
  - Infiltration into the surrounding pericolonic fat can indicate extension of tumor outside of the colonic serosa and local invasion
  - Retroperitoneal lymph nodes or pelvic nodes greater than 1 cm in the short axis, or clusters of intra-abdominal nodes may indicate regional lymph node metastases

FIGURE 8.6 A,B

A. Psoas muscle
B. Small bowel loops
C. Vertebra
D. Liver
E. Portal vein
F. Right common iliac artery
G. Stomach
H. Spleen
I. Bladder

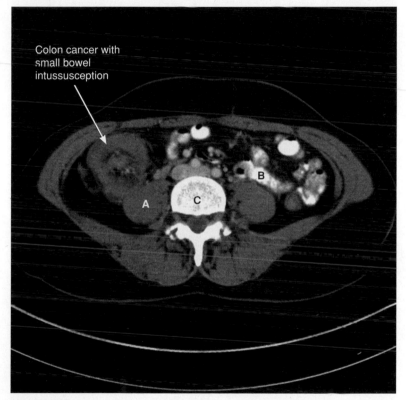

Colon cancer with small bowel intussusception

FIGURE 8.6 A

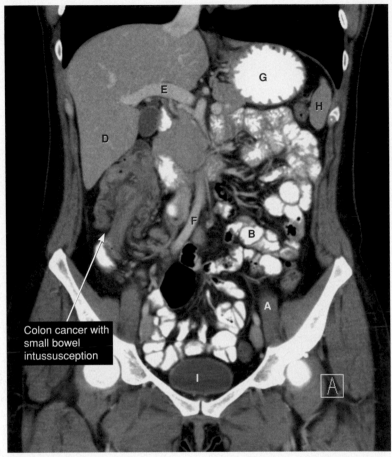

Colon cancer with small bowel intussusception

FIGURE 8.6 B

Rectal Cancer

- **EUS findings**
  - Has better differentiation of wall layers than MRI
  - Useful in the assessment of early tumor involvement

- **CT findings** (Fig. 8.7)
  - Soft tissue mass within/around the rectum
- **MRI findings**
  - Helpful to determine need for chemoradiation therapy through visualization of tumor involvement of the mesorectal fascia
  - Extramural spread, fascial involvement, and peritoneal infiltration can be seen best with high resolution rectal imaging
  - T1- and T2-weighted images under high resolution can visualize extent of disease

FIGURE 8.7 A,B

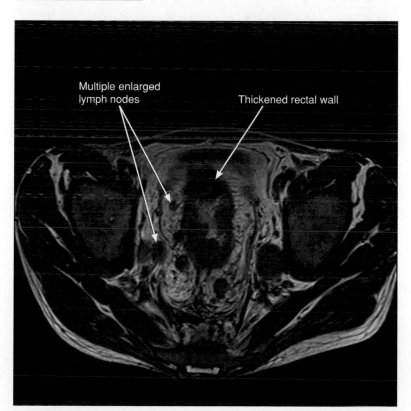

Multiple enlarged lymph nodes

Thickened rectal wall

FIGURE 8.7 A

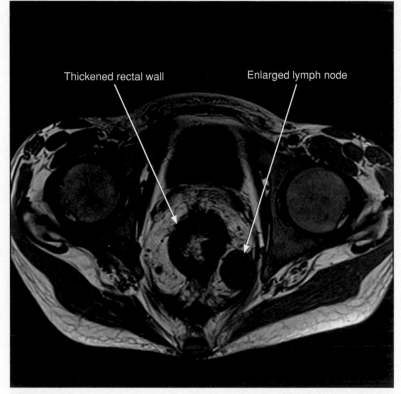

Thickened rectal wall   Enlarged lymph node

FIGURE 8.7 B

Volvulus

Overview

- Due to twisting of the bowel around its mesentery
- Sigmoid (80% to 90%) > cecal (10%) > transverse colon (rare)

Signs and Symptoms

- Abdominal pain, nausea, vomiting, abdominal distension

Diagnosis

- Plain films (details in radiology section)
  - Sigmoid volvulus: Classic findings—bent inner tube or inverted U in the right upper quadrant, bird beak's sign
  - Cecal volvulus: Classic findings—coffee bean sign with cecum in the left upper quadrant
- CT imaging: Whirl sign (vessels swirling around each other when scrolling through the abdomen)

Treatment

- Sigmoid volvulus: Possible endoscopic decompression then elective sigmoidectomy
  - If physical examination is negative for diffuse peritonitis: Colonoscopic decompression or barium enema followed by elective sigmoidectomy during the same hospitalization
  - If physical examination is positive for diffuse peritonitis: Surgical exploration, Hartman's procedure vs. sigmoidectomy with primary anastomosis
- Cecal volvulus: Exploratory laparotomy, cecectomy, or right hemicolectomy

RADIOLOGY

Sigmoid Volvulus

- **Plain film findings** (Fig. 8.8)
  - "Bird's beak" twist may be seen
  - Absent haustral folds within an inverted U-shaped loop that is massively distended
  - The apex of the inverted U-shaped loop lies high in the abdomen above the level of T10
- **CT findings** (Fig. 8.8)
  - Whirling of the twisted mesentery involved with the sigmoid volvulus can be seen

FIGURE 8.8 A–G

A. Psoas muscle   D. Portal vein
B. Vertebra   E. Bladder
C. Liver

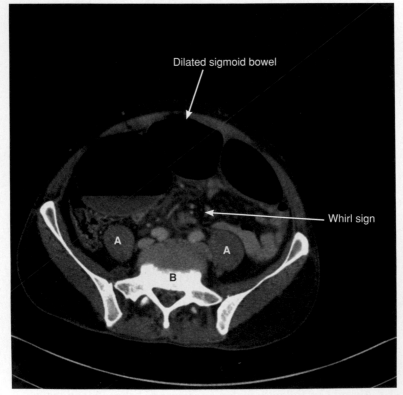

FIGURE 8.8 A

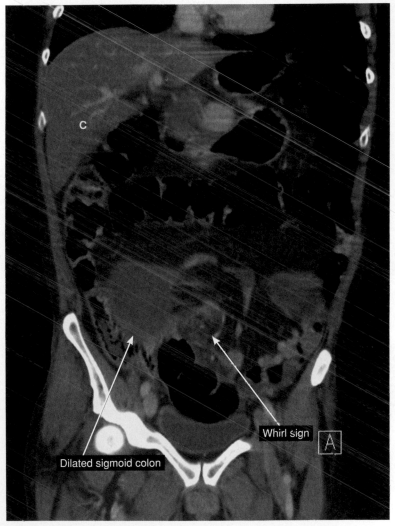

FIGURE 8.8 B

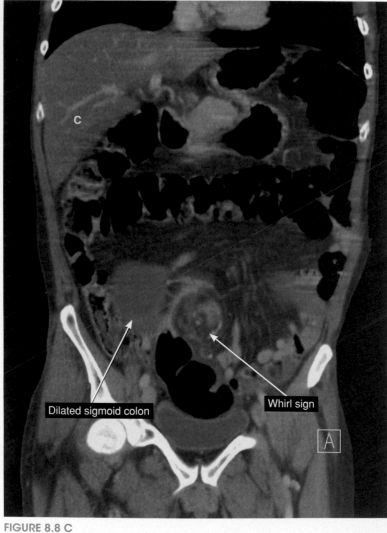

FIGURE 8.8 C

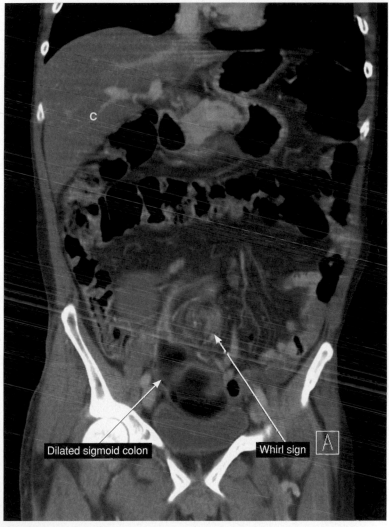

FIGURE 8.8 D

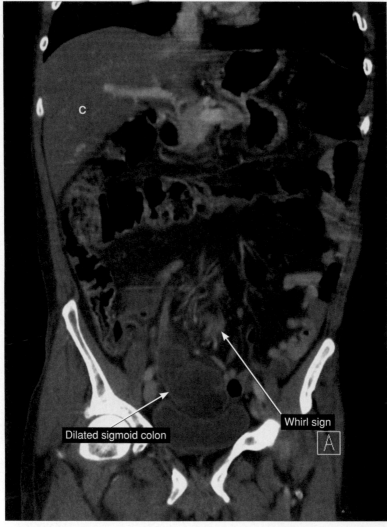

FIGURE 8.8 E

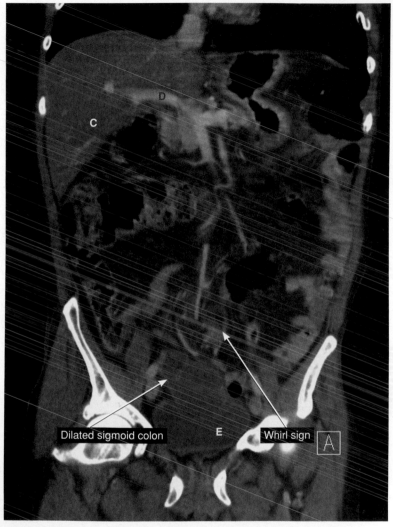

FIGURE 8.8 F

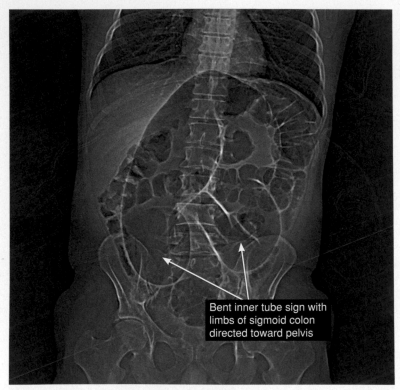

Bent inner tube sign with limbs of sigmoid colon directed toward pelvis

FIGURE 8.8 G

Cecal Volvulus

■ **Plain film findings**
  • "Bird's beak"-type twist or coffee bean sign may be seen
  • In half of the cecal volvulus cases, the cecum twists and inverts such that pole of the cecum and appendix occupy the left upper quadrant; whereas in the other half of the cases, the dilated cecum can be anywhere within the abdomen

■ **CT findings** (Fig. 8.9)
  • Twisted bowel and mesentery is seen as a "whirl sign" and is proportional to the degree of rotation

FIGURE 8.9 A–D

A. Sacrum
B. Ilium
C. Small bowel loops
D. Psoas muscle
E. Liver
F. Kidney
G. Stomach
H. Spleen
I. Vertebra
J. IVC
K. Bladder

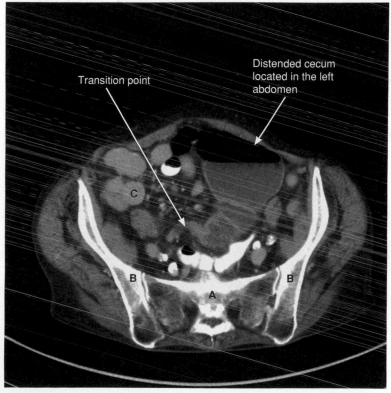

FIGURE 8.9 A

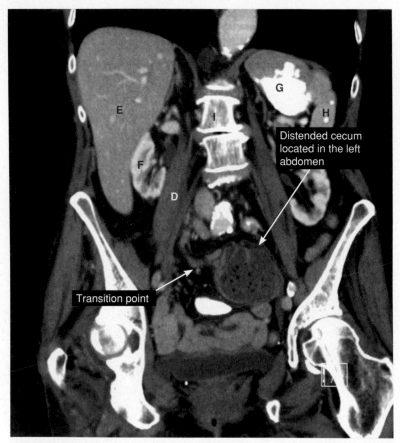

Distended cecum located in the left abdomen

Transition point

FIGURE 8.9 B

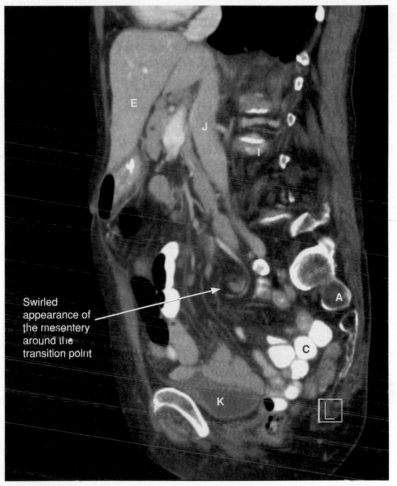

Swirled appearance of the mesentery around the transition point

FIGURE 8.9 C

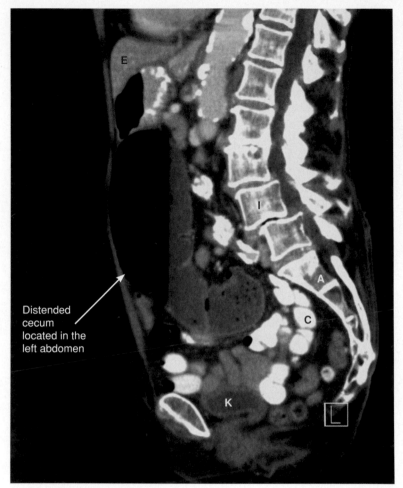

Distended cecum located in the left abdomen

FIGURE 8.9 D

Perirectal Abscess

Overview

- Initial infection from an obstructed anal gland, leading to abscess collection in the potential space around the anus and rectum
- Perirectal abscess are classified according to their location: Perianal abscess, ischiorectal abscess, intersphincteric abscess, supralevator abscess, and deep postanal space abscess

Signs and Symptoms

- Usually based on physical examination: Severe pain upon palpation, may have an area of redness, swelling, and fluctuance in the involved region
- Patients may have fever, urinary retention, leukocytosis

Diagnosis

- Usually based on physical examination. However, deeper abscess may require examination under anesthesia or further imaging such as MRI of the pelvis or transanal ultrasonography

Treatment

- Surgical drainage is the usual treatment
- Horseshoe abscess require concurrent drainage of the deep postanal space

RADIOLOGY

Perirectal Abscess

- **CT/MRI findings** (Fig. 8.10)
  - Gas-containing fluid collections in the perirectal region with surrounding fat stranding

FIGURE 8.10 A,B

A. Rectum
B. Corpus cavernosum
C. Femur

D. Adductor magnus
E. Gluteus maximus

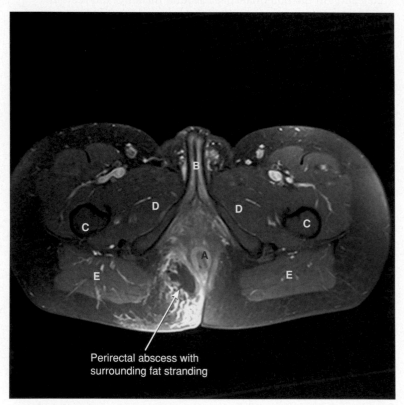

Perirectal abscess with surrounding fat stranding

FIGURE 8.10 A

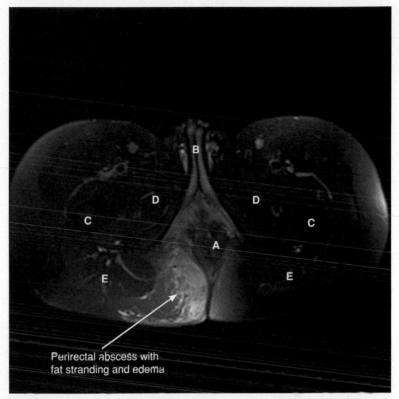

Perirectal abscess with
fat stranding and edema

FIGURE 8.10 B

Horseshoe Abscess

- **CT findings**
  - Rim-enhancing, fluid collection in the shape of a "U" near the rectum
- **MRI findings** (Fig. 8.11)
  - T2-weighted image shows a hyperintense fluid collection in the shape of a "U" encircling the rectum

FIGURE 8.11

A. Rectum   C. Ischial tuberosity

B. Pubic symphysis   D. Corpus cavernosum

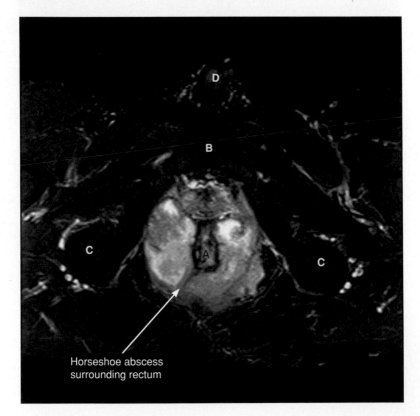

Horseshoe abscess surrounding rectum

Ogilvie's Syndrome

Overview

- Also known as acute colonic pseudo-obstruction
- A functional disorder without any mechanical obstruction

Signs and Symptoms

- Abdominal distention without flatus or bowel movement over several days
- Usually occurs in elderly patients who has had prolonged hospitalization or in patients who are on significant amounts of narcotics

Diagnosis

- Serial abdominal x-rays and abdominal physical examination

Treatment/Management

- Bowel rest, IV hydration, correct underlying electrolyte abnormalities, discontinue narcotics, and anticholinergics
- If conservative treatment fails, neostigmine (acetylcholinesterase inhibitor) IV push over 2 to 3 minutes
  - Monitor for bradycardia
- Colonoscopic decompression

> KEY POINT
>
> - Cecum greater than 12 cm is at risk for ischemia and cecum greater than 14 cm is at risk for perforation

RADIOLOGY

Ogilvie's Syndrome

- **Plain film findings** (Fig. 8.12)
  - Dilated large bowel loops throughout the abdomen, sometimes with air-fluid levels
- **CT findings** (Fig. 8.12)
  - Marked, diffuse colonic dilation without an obstructing lesion

FIGURE 8.12 A–C

A. Psoas muscle C. Small bowel loops
B. Vertebra D. Liver

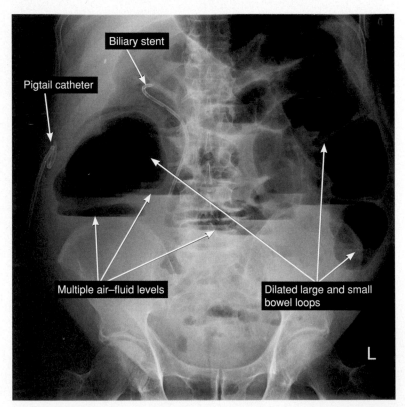

FIGURE 8.12 A

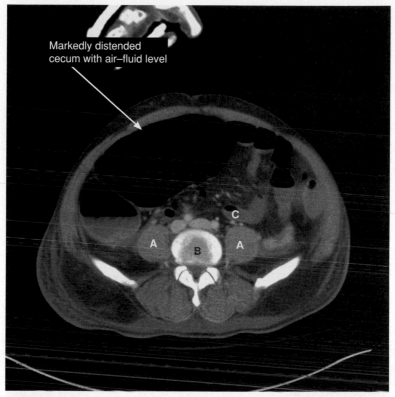

Markedly distended cecum with air–fluid level

FIGURE 8.12 B

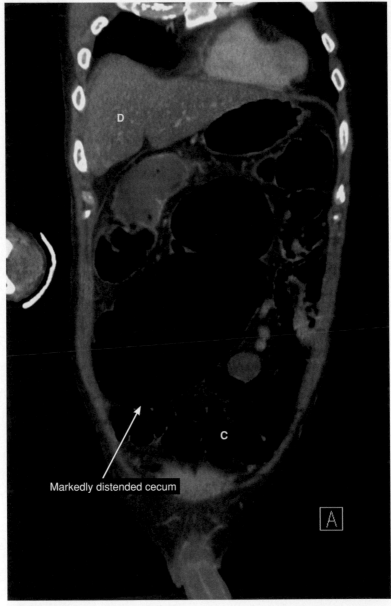

FIGURE 8.12 C

Suggested Readings

Batke M, Cappell MS. Adynamic ileus and acute colonic pseudo-obstruction. *Med Clin North Am.* 2008;92(3):649–670.

Beets-Tan RG, Beets GL. Rectal cancer: Review with emphasis on MR imaging. *Radiology.* 2004;232(2):335–346.

Beets-Tan RG, Beets GL, van der Hoop AG, et al. Preoperative MR imaging of anal fistulas: Does it really help the surgeon? *Radiology.* 2001;218(1):75–84.

Brunicardi FC, Andersen DK, Billiar TR, et al. *Schwartz's Principles of Surgery*, 9th ed. New York, NY: McGraw-Hill; 2010:1013–1072.

Chintapalli KN, Chopra S, Ghiatas AA, et al. Diverticulitis versus colon cancer: Differentiation with helical CT findings. *Radiology.* 1999;210(2):429–435.

Choi JS, Lim JS, Kim H, et al. Colonic pseudoobstruction: CT findings. *AJR Am J Roentgenol.* 2008;190(6):1521–1526.

Engel AF, Eijsbouts Q. Horseshoe ischiorectal abscess originating from dorsal intersphincteric cryptoglandular abscess. *J Am Coll Surg.* 2001;192(5):664.

Feig BW, Ching CD. *The MD Anderson Surgical Oncology Handbook*, 5th ed. Philadelphia, PA: Lippincott Williams & Wilkins; 2012:347–397.

Furukawa A, Kanasaki S, Kono N, et al. CT diagnosis of acute mesenteric ischemia from various causes. *AJR Am J Roentgenol.* 2009;192(2):408–416.

Goldman SM, Fishman EK, Gatewood OM, et al. CT in the diagnosis of enterovesical fistulae. *AJR Am J Roentgenol.* 1985;144(6):1229–1233.

Horton KM, Abrams RA, Fishman EK. Spiral CT of colon cancer: Imaging features and role in management. *Radiographics.* 2000;20(2):419–430.

Horton KM, Corl FM, Fishman EK. CT evaluation of the colon: Inflammatory disease. *Radiographics.* 2000;20(2):399–418.

Klingensmith ME, Aziz A, Bharat A, et al. *The Washington Manual of Surgery*, 6th ed. Philadelphia, PA: Lippincott Williams & Wilkins; 2012:303–305.

Levsky JM, Den EI, DuBrow RA, et al. CT findings of sigmoid volvulus. *AJR Am J Roentgenol.* 2010;194(1):136–143.

Madiba TE, Thomson SR. The management of cecal volvulus. *Dis Colon Rectum.* 2002;45(2):264–267.

Maykel JA, Opelka FG. Colonic diverticulosis and diverticular hemorrhage. *Clin Colon Rectal Surg.* 2004;17(3):195–204.

Osiro SB, Cunningham D, Shoja MM, et al. The twisted colon: A review of sigmoid volvulus. *Am Surg.* 2012;78(3):271–279.

Ponec RJ, Saunders MD, Kimmey MB. Neostigmine for the treatment of acute colonic pseudo-obstruction. *N Engl J Med.* 1999;341(3):137–141.

Rosen SA, Colguhoun P, Efron J, et.al. Horseshoe abscesses and fistulas: How are we doing? *Surg Innov.* 2006;13(1):17–21.

Rosenblat JM, Rozenblit AM, Wolf EL, et al. Findings of cecal volvulus at CT. *Radiology.* 2010;256(1):169–175.

Siewert B, Tye G, Kruskal J, et al. Impact of CT-guided drainage in the treatment of diverticular abscesses: Size matters. *AJR Am J Roentgenol.* 2006;186(3):680–686.

Stoker J, Rociu E, Zwamborn AW, et al. Endoluminal MR imaging of the rectum and anus: Technique, applications, and pitfalls. *Radiographics.* 1999;19(2):383–398.

Stollman N, Raskin JB. Diverticular disease of the colon. *Lancet.* 2004;363(9409):631–639.

Townsend CM, Beauchamp RD, Evers BM, et.al. *Sabiston Textbook of Surgery: The Biological Basis of Modern Surgical Practice*, 19th ed. Philadelphia, PA: Elsevier Saunders; 2012.

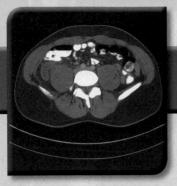

9

Appendix

Appendicitis

Overview

- Most common in teenage years and patients in their 20s
- Rate of appendectomy for appendicitis is 10 per 10,000 patients per year
- Usually due to lymphoid hyperplasia or fecalith causing luminal obstruction

Signs and Symptoms

- Anorexia (90%)
- Abdominal pain: Periumbilical migrating to RLQ
- Nausea and vomiting (70%)
- Low-grade fever

Physical Examination Findings

- Point tenderness typically over McBurney point
- Psoas sign: Pain with extension of right thigh while in left lateral decubitus position
- Obturator sign: Pain with passive rotation of flexed right hip
- Rovsing's sign: Pain in RLQ while palpating LLQ
- Rectal examination may reveal a pelvic mass or abscess

Laboratory Findings

- Patients can have a normal WBC count, but usually mild leukocytosis in the range of 10,000 to 18,000/mm^3
- Urinalysis may be positive with pyuria, hematuria, and albuminuria

Treatment

- IV fluid resuscitation and peri-operative antibiotics
- Laparoscopic or open appendectomy
- For perforated appendix, may undergo appendectomy if there is no inflammatory phlegmon. If there is an inflammatory phlegmon, conservative management with IV antibiotic, with percutaneous drainage of any associated abscess

---

KEY POINT

- The risk of a ruptured appendicitis increases at 24 hours from the initial presentation of signs and symptoms

---

RADIOLOGY

Appendicitis

- **Plain film findings**
  - Usually normal
  - Adynamic ileus may be seen
  - Sometimes, a calcified appendicolith in the right lower quadrant is seen
- **US findings**
  - Blind-ending tubular structure that is noncompressible, outer wall to outer wall diameter greater than 6 mm
  - If identified, an appendicolith casts a clean posterior acoustic shadow
  - Tenderness over appendix
  - False negative can result from retrocecal appendicitis, gangrenous or perforated appendicitis, gas-filled appendix, and massively enlarged appendix
- **CT findings** (Fig. 9.1)
  - Appendix measuring greater than 6 mm in diameter, failure of appendix to fill with oral contrast or air up to its tip
  - Adjacent cecal thickening due to edema at the origin of the appendix

- Inflammation/fatty stranding/fluid in the retroperitoneum/frank abscess
- Appendicolith
- **MRI findings**
  - Dilated, thickened appendix with adjacent inflammation seen on contrast-enhanced T1-weighted and T2-weighted images

FIGURE 9.1 A,B

A. Vertebra
B. Psoas muscle
C. Colon

D. Stomach
E. Spleen
F. Bladder

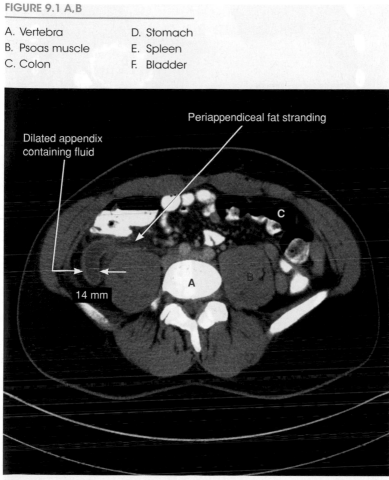

FIGURE 9.1 A

FIGURE 9.2 A,B

A. Femoral head   D. Small bowel loops
B. Liver   E. Colon
C. Stomach

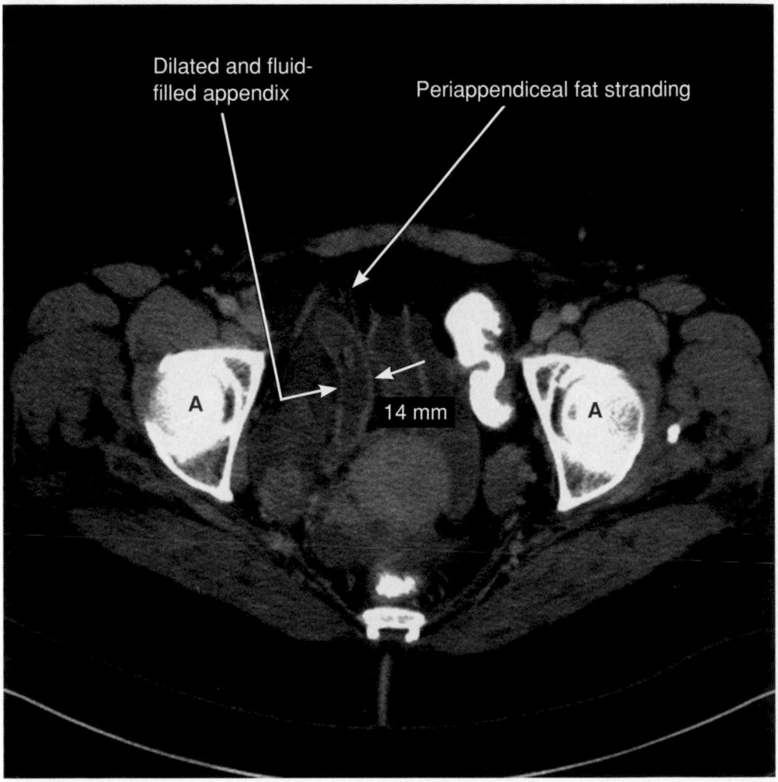

FIGURE 9.2 A

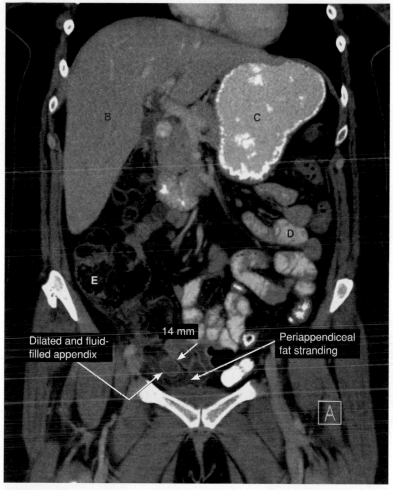

FIGURE 9.2 B

Appendicitis with Appendicolith

- **US findings**
  - Echogenic mass noted within the appendiceal lumen, usually with dense posterior acoustic shadowing
- **CT findings** (Fig. 9.3)
  - Enlarged appendix with a hyperdense mass within the lumen

FIGURE 9.3 A–C

A. Small bowel loops	D. Gallbladder
B. Liver	E. Spleen
C. Stomach	

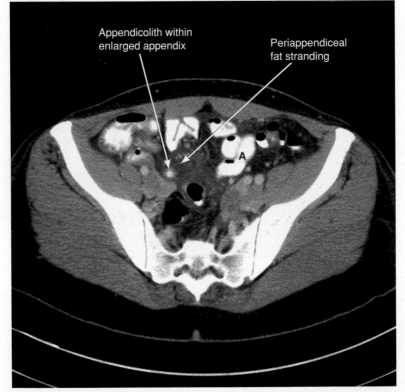

Appendicolith within enlarged appendix

Periappendiceal fat stranding

FIGURE 9.3 A

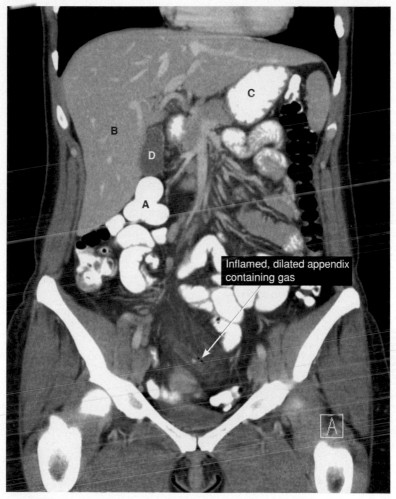

Inflamed, dilated appendix containing gas

FIGURE 9.3 B

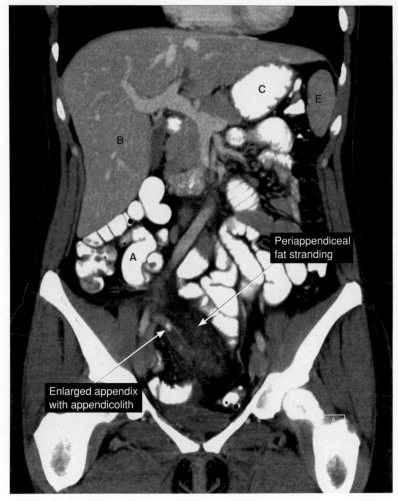

FIGURE 9.3 C

Enlarged Appendix

- **CT findings** (Fig. 9.4)
  - Appendix measuring greater than 6 mm in diameter without evidence of inflammation

FIGURE 9.4 A,B

A. Vertebra   D. Liver
B. Psoas muscle   E. Stomach
C. Small bowel loops

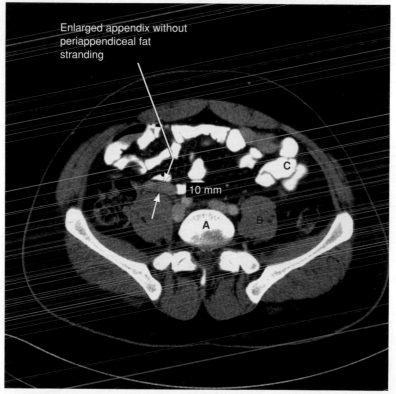

Enlarged appendix without periappendiceal fat stranding

10 mm

FIGURE 9.4 A

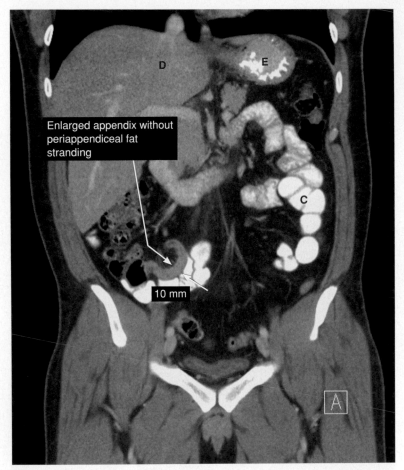

Enlarged appendix without periappendiceal fat stranding

10 mm

FIGURE 9.4 B

Residual Appendix

- **CT findings** (Fig. 9.5)
  - Remaining base of appendix with appendiceal wall thickening and periappendiceal fat stranding

FIGURE 9.5 A–C

A. Vertebra   D. Liver

B. Psoas muscle   E. Stomach

C. Small bowel loops F. Bladder

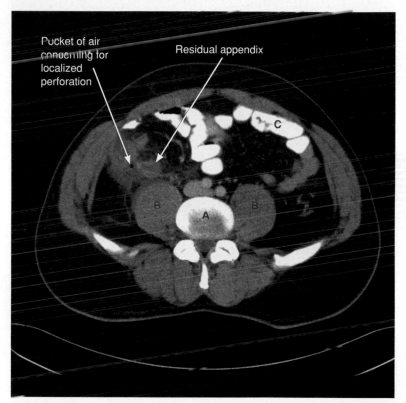

FIGURE 9.5 A

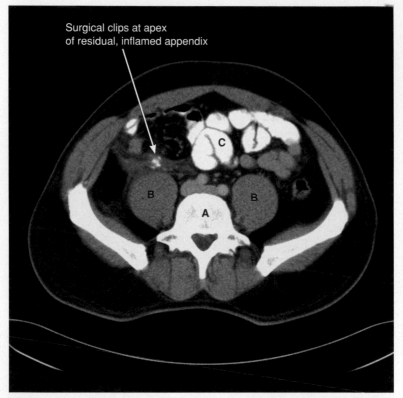

Surgical clips at apex
of residual, inflamed appendix

FIGURE 9.5 B

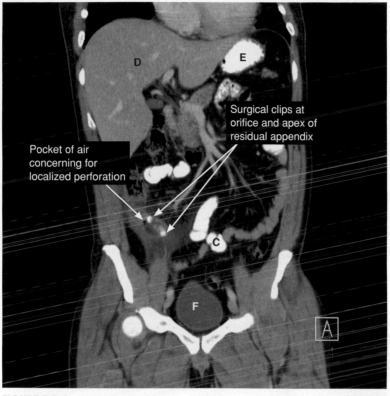

Pocket of air
concerning for
localized perforation

Surgical clips at
orifice and apex of
residual appendix

FIGURE 9.5 C

Ruptured Appendix with Abscess

- **Plain film findings**
  - Abscess may indent the medial border of the cecum
- **US findings**
  - Rim enhancing fluid collection seen around the appendix with phlegmon
- **CT findings** (Fig. 9.6)
  - Fluid collection adjacent to an inflamed appendix with periappendiceal fat stranding

FIGURE 9.6 A–D

A. Small bowel loops	D. Liver
B. Bladder	E. Stomach
C. Rectum	F. Vertebra

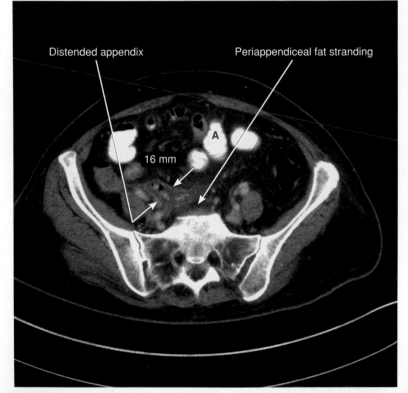

Distended appendix   Periappendiceal fat stranding

16 mm

FIGURE 9.6 A

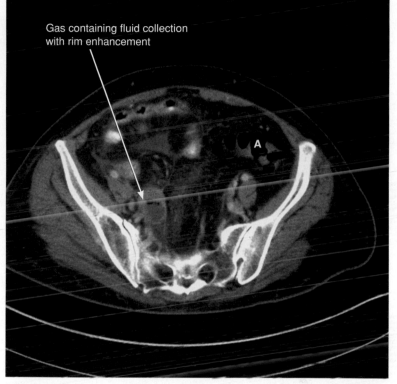

Gas containing fluid collection with rim enhancement

A

FIGURE 9.6 B

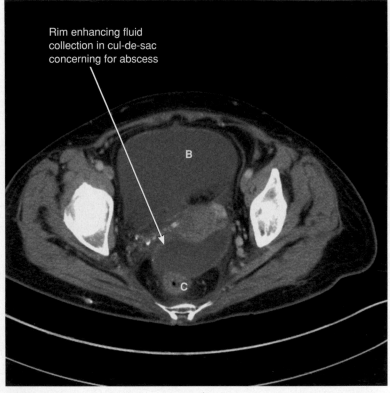

Rim enhancing fluid collection in cul-de-sac concerning for abscess

FIGURE 9.6 C

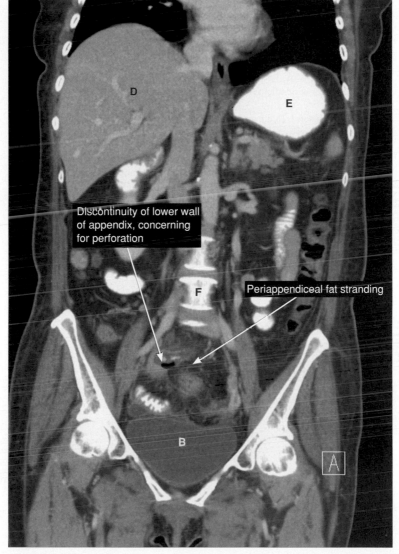

Discontinuity of lower wall of appendix, concerning for perforation

Periappendiceal fat stranding

FIGURE 9.6 D

Suggested Readings

Birnbaum BA, Wilson SR. Appendicitis at the millennium. *Radiology.* 2000;215: 337–348.

Cartwright SL, Knudson MP. Evaluation of acute abdominal pain in adults. *Am Fam Physician.* 2008;77(7):971–978.

Hlibczuk V, Dattaro JA, Jin Z, et al. Diagnostic accuracy of noncontrast computed tomography for appendicitis in adults: A systematic review. *Ann Emerg Med.* 2010; 55(1):51–59.

Humes DJ, Simpson J. Acute appendicitis. *BMJ.* 2006;333(7567):530–534.

Lowe LH, Penney MW, Scheker LE, et al. Appendicolith revealed on CT in children with suspected appendicitis: How specific is it in the diagnosis of appendicitis? *AJR Am J Roentgenol.* 2000;175:981–984.

Morrow SE, Newman KD. Current management of appendicitis. *Semin Pediatr Surg.* 2007;16:34–40.

Prystowsky JB, Pugh CM, Nagle AP. Current problems in surgery. Appendicitis. *Curr Probl Surg.* 2005;42(10):688–742.

Shin LK, Halpern D, Weston SR, et al. Prospective CT diagnosis of stump appendicitis. *AJR Am J Roentgenol.* 2005;184:S62–S64.

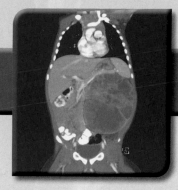

10

Kidney

Renal Cyst

Overview

- Usually benign and found in population over the age of 50 years

Signs and Symptoms

- Usually asymptomatic and incidentally found on imaging

Diagnosis

- CT, ultrasound, or MRI

Treatment

- Majority do not require treatment
- Percutaneous drainage for symptomatic benign cysts
- Partial or total nephrectomy for complex cystic lesions suspicious of malignancy

The Bosniak Classification for Renal Cysts

- Category I

  Simple cyst without septa, calcifications, or solid components. Cyst does not enhance on imaging. Risk of malignancy 0% to <2%

- Category II

  Cyst with a few thin septa. There might be presence of fine calcifications within the septa or wall. Cysts are <3 cm in size, well marginated. Cyst does not enhance on imaging. Risk of malignancy 13%

- Category IIF

  Cyst may contain more thin septa but the septa or wall does not enhance on imaging. Cyst might contain thicker or even nodular calcifications that does not enhance on imaging. There are no enhancing soft tissue elements. Lesions that are intrarenal, measuring ≥3 cm without enhancement on imaging are also included in this category. Risk of malignancy 14% to 24%

- Category III

  Indeterminate cystic lesions with thickened, irregular wall or septa. Positive enhancement on imaging. Risk of malignancy 50%

- Category IV

  Complex cystic lesions that have all the characteristics under category III. Also, the lesion has adjacent enhancing soft tissue component which is independent of the wall or septa. Risk of malignancy 90%

RADIOLOGY

- **US findings**
  - Anechoic, well-defined masses, with thin walls and posterior acoustic enhancement
- **CT findings** (Fig. 10.1)
  - Well-defined rounded mass with low attenuation values of 0 to 20 HU

- Well defined walls with or without septae (refer to Bosniak classification)
- No internal enhancement on post contrast images
- **MRI findings**
  - Well defined lesion usually with low signal intensity on T1-weighted images if it contains simple fluid, or higher signal intensity if it contains blood
  - Uniformly hyperintense on T2-weighted images
  - No internal enhancement after contrast medium administration

FIGURE 10.1 A–C

A. Vertebra   E. Liver
B. Descending aorta   F. Stomach
C. IVC   G. Spleen
D. Small bowel loops   H. Psoas muscle

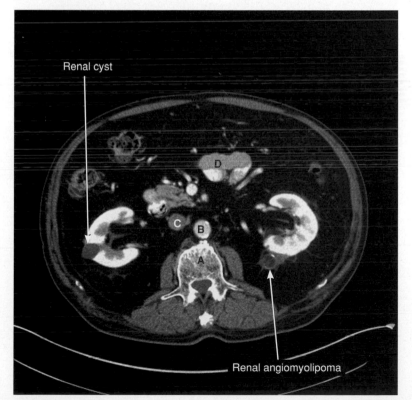

FIGURE 10.1 A

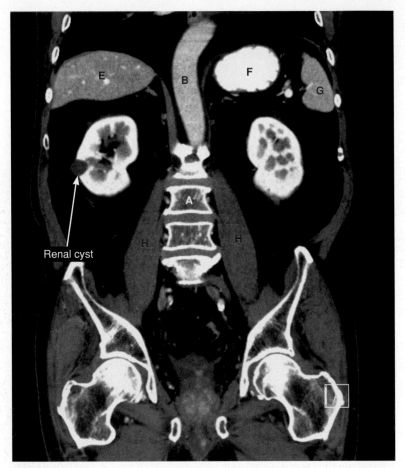

FIGURE 10.1 B

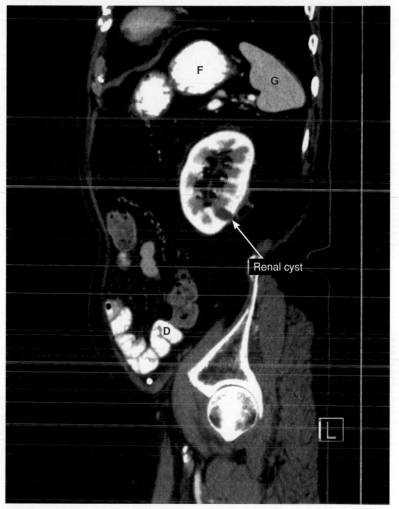

FIGURE 10.1 C

Renal Cell Carcinoma

Overview

- Most common kidney cancer in the adult population
- Most are found incidentally on radiology imaging
- Most common in men ages 50 to 70 years of age
- Risk factors include smoking and obesity

Clinical Presentation

- Flank pain, hematuria, palpable flank mass (10% of patients have this triad)
- Weight loss
- Common sites of metastasis are lung, bone, and liver

Diagnosis

- Obtain a noncontrast study and a contrast study to look for increased enhancement of the mass after injection of contrast
- If patient cannot receive contrast, consider an MRI with gadolinium, if GFR (glomerular filtration rate) > 30
- CXR or Chest CT to rule out metastasis

Treatment

- After appropriate staging is made, then perform radical or partial nephrectomy depending on the size or location of the tumor
- Possibly requires immunotherapy such as interleukin-2 or interferon alpha

RADIOLOGY

- **Plain film findings**
  - Often normal unless mass is large or contains calcification
  - Mass effects on nearby organs may be seen if tumor is very large

- **CT findings** (Fig. 10.2)
  - Enhancement pattern may be heterogeneous due to the presence of hemorrhage and/or necrosis
  - Detection of small hypervascular RCC masses is optimal in the corticomedullary or nephrographic phase
  - RCC usually shows a lobular margin with adjacent normal tissue but can sometimes infiltrate calyces or the renal pelvis
  - Tumor spread through the renal veins and into the IVC may warrant cardiopulmonary bypass if tumor resection is elected
- **MRI findings**
  - Renal cell carcinomas demonstrate contrast enhancement on T1-weight images, and variable signal characteristics on T2-weighted images

FIGURE 10.2 A,B

A. Kidney
B. Vertebra
C. Descending aorta
D. IVC
E. Transverse colon
F. Small bowel loops
G. Liver
H. Stomach
I. Spleen

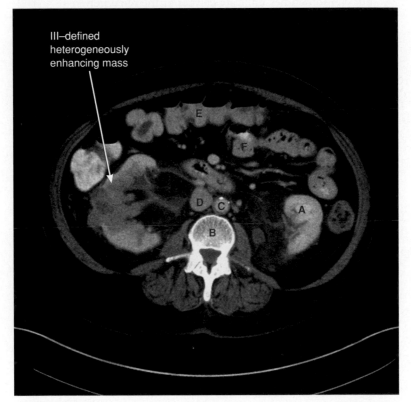

Ill–defined heterogeneously enhancing mass

FIGURE 10.2 A

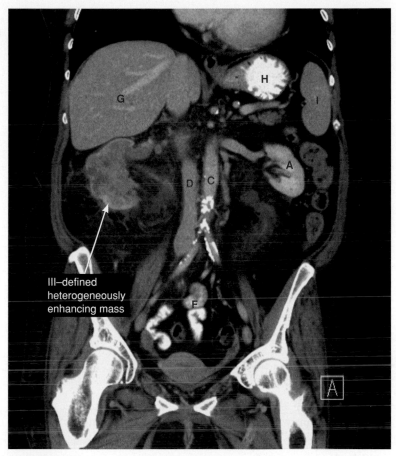

FIGURE 10.2 B

Wilms Tumor

Overview

- Most common malignant kidney tumor in childhood (age 2 to 4 years)
- Associated with WAGR syndrome: **W**ilms tumor, **A**niridia, **G**enitourinary malformation, mental **R**etardation

Signs and Symptoms

- Nausea, vomiting, hematuria, abdominal distension from mass effect

Diagnosis

- Chest and abdominal CT to characterize the tumor
- Ultrasound to evaluate the vasculature in preparation for surgical resection

Treatment

- Surgical resection, possible chemotherapy based on staging

RADIOLOGY

- **Plain film findings**
  - Displacement of abdominal viscera may be seen
  - Calcifications within the mass can be seen in a minority of cases
  - Often large at presentation and commonly cross the midline
- **US findings**
  - Usually heterogeneous at presentation with or without associated retroperitoneal hemorrhage
  - Calcification is uncommon
  - Contralateral kidney should always be examined due to increased risk of bilaterality
- **CT findings** (Fig. 10.3)
  - Large, heterogeneously enhancing mass arising from the kidney parenchyma
  - Distortion of renal collecting system
  - Metastases to the liver and lungs may be seen

- **MRI findings**
  - Heterogeneously enhancing mass arising from the kidney on T1-weighted images, and variable signal characteristics on T2-weighted images

FIGURE 10.3 A,B

A. Vertebra   D. Colon
B. Kidney   E. Bladder
C. Liver

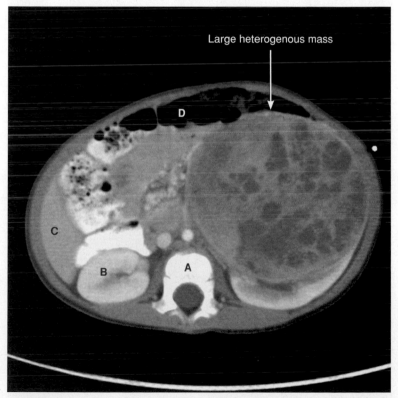

FIGURE 10.3 A

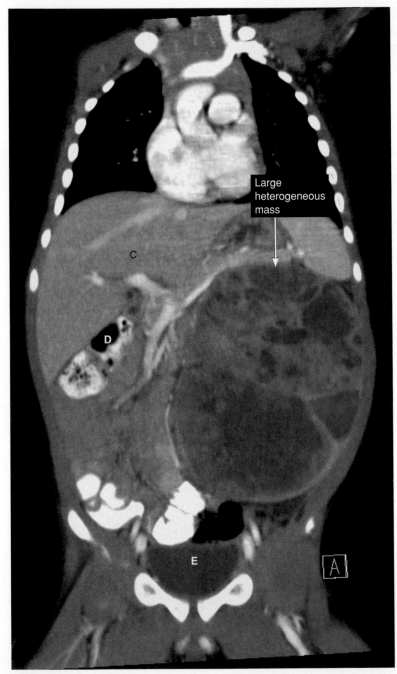

FIGURE 10.3 B

Horseshoe Kidney

- Congenital partial or complete fusion of the kidney inferior to the inferior mesenteric artery
- Usually asymptomatic but patients are more susceptible to kidney stones and infection
- Patients also have an increased risk for kidney cancer

RADIOLOGY

- **Plain film findings**
  - Lower position of both renal shadows
  - Lower pole calyces lie closer to the spine, usually medially rotated, and may lie medial to the ureters
- **US findings**
  - Isthmus connecting the lower poles
  - Altered renal axis of both kidneys
  - Hypoechoic soft tissue mass anterior to the spine
- **CT findings** (Fig. 10.4)
  - Fused kidneys located below the origin of the inferior mesenteric artery
  - Malrotated collecting system may be seen
  - Multiple renal arteries with aberrant origins from the aorta
- **MRI findings**
  - Fused kidneys located below the origin of the inferior mesenteric artery

FIGURE 10.4 A,B

A. Air within stomach
B. Small bowel loops
C. Psoas muscle
D. Vertebra

E. Descending aorta
F. Stomach
G. Liver

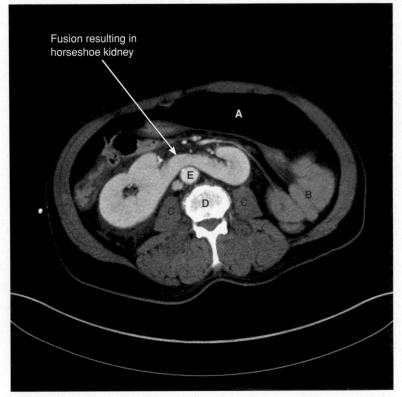

Fusion resulting in horseshoe kidney

FIGURE 10.4 A

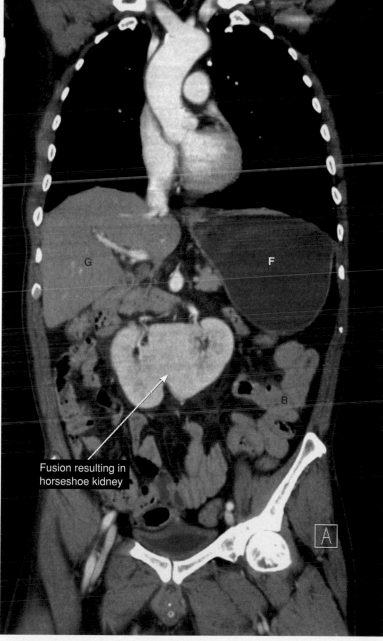

Fusion resulting in horseshoe kidney

FIGURE 10.4 B

Suggested Readings

Aquisto TM, Yost R, Marshall KW. Best cases from the AFIP: Anaplastic Wilms tumor: Radiologic and pathologic findings. *Radiographics.* 2004;24:1709–1713.

Dyer RB, Chen MY, Zagoria RJ. Classic signs in uroradiology. *Radiographics.* 2004;24:S247–S280.

Israel GM, Hindman N, Bosniak MA. Evaluation of cystic renal masses: Comparison of CT and MR imaging by using the Bosniak classification system. *Radiology.* 2004;231:365–371.

Sheth S, Scatarige JC, Horton KM, et al. Current concepts in the diagnosis and management of renal cell carcinoma: Role of multidetector CT and three-dimensional CT. *Radiographics.* 2001;21:S237–S254.

Slywotzky CM, Bosniak MA. Localized cystic disease of the kidney. *AJR Am J Roentgenol.* 2001;176(4):843–849.

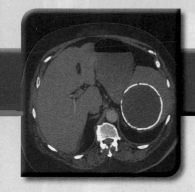

11

Spleen

Splenic Artery Aneurysm

Overview

- Most common visceral artery aneurysm
- Third most common intra-abdominal aneurysm after abdominal aortic aneurysm and iliac artery aneurysm
- Risk factors include collagen vascular disorder, portal hypertension, pregnancy, trauma, pancreatitis, and fibrodysplasia

Signs and Symptoms

- Mostly asymptomatic
- May have vague left upper quadrant or epigastric pain
- If ruptured, patient will display signs of hypovolemic shock along with abdominal distension

Diagnosis

- CT angiography, MRI/MRA, or abdominal ultrasound

Treatment/Management

- Operative management if ≥2 cm, pregnancy, anticipated pregnancy, pseudoaneurysm, expanding aneurysm, or if patient is symptomatic
- Operative management includes aneurysmectomy, partial splenectomy, endovascular embolization, or stent graft exclusion of the aneurysm

RADIOLOGY

- **Plain film findings**
  - Splenic artery calcifications may be seen in the left upper quadrant
- **CT findings** (Fig. 11.1)
  - Focal dilation of the splenic artery, usually containing wall calcifications
  - Enhancement equal to that of the aorta
  - May contain mural thrombus

FIGURE 11.1 A–F

A. Liver   D. Descending aorta
B. Kidney   E. Vertebra
C. Spleen

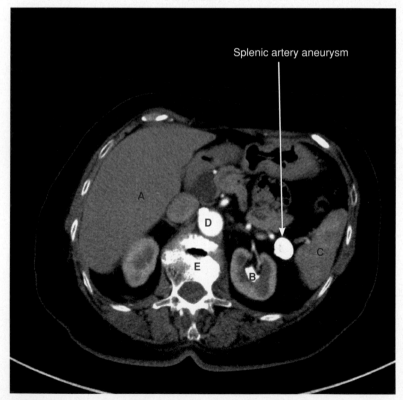

FIGURE 11.1 A

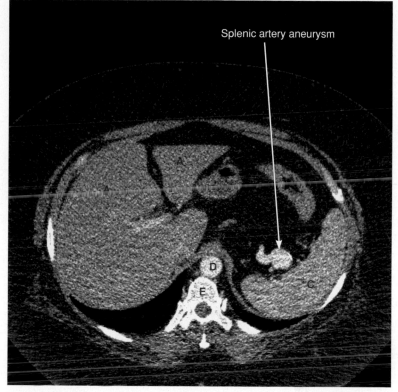

Splenic artery aneurysm

FIGURE 11.1 B

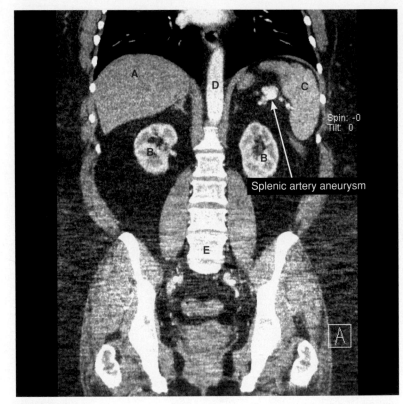

FIGURE 11.1 C

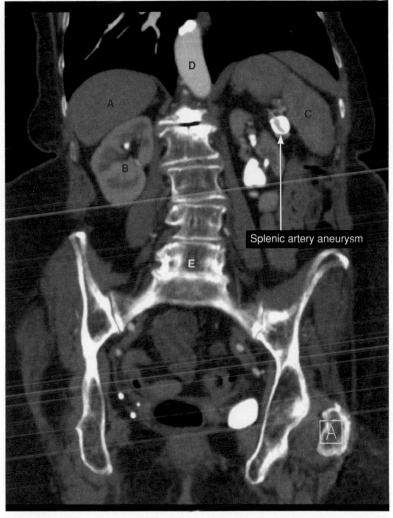

Splenic artery aneurysm

FIGURE 11.1 D

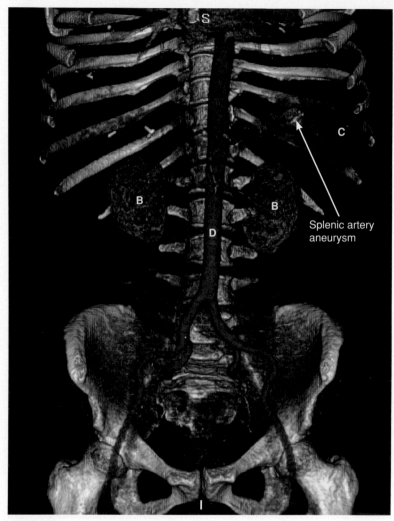

FIGURE 11.1 E

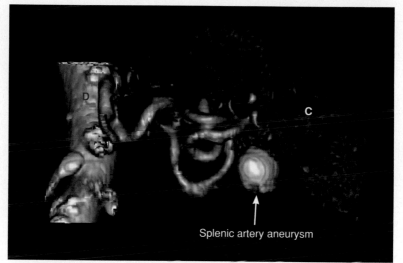

Splenic artery aneurysm

FIGURE 11.1 F

Splenic Cyst

Overview

- Categorized into the following:
  - Nonparasitic cyst (two types):
    - Congenital—true epidermoid cyst (has an epithelial lining)
    - Pseudocyst—acquired from trauma
  - Parasitic cyst: From echinococcal infection

Signs and Symptoms

- Typically asymptomatic and found incidentally
- If cyst is large enough, patient will experience abdominal pain with left-sided scapular or shoulder pain, early satiety, nausea or vomiting, weight loss

Diagnosis

- Ultrasound—can establish the presence of a cystic lesion
- CT—nonenhancing cystic lesion within the spleen
- Peripheral or septal calcifications may be seen
- Serology for echinococcal antibodies

Treatment/Management

- Nonparasitic cysts
  - Asymptomatic—observation
  - Symptomatic—unroofing, partial splenectomy
- Parasitic cyst—splenectomy
  - Avoid spillage of cyst contents intraoperatively (results in anaphylactic shock)

RADIOLOGY

- **Plain film findings** (Fig. 11.2 D)
  - May see a calcifications outlining the cyst
- **US findings** (Fig. 11.2 E)
  - Pseudocysts may show internal echoes from debris
  - Pseudocysts may show echogenic foci with posterior acoustic shadowing due to calcification
- **CT findings** (Fig. 11.2 A,B,C)
  - Homogeneous, well-circumscribed, fluid attenuation
  - No internal enhancement
  - Cyst wall calcification may be present
  - May contain internal septations
- **MRI findings**
  - Homogeneous, well-circumscribed, T2 hyperintense due to fluid
  - Pseudocysts have variable signal intensity on T1-weighted images due to the presence of blood or proteinaceous material

FIGURE 11.2 A–E

A. Liver   E. Psoas muscle
B. Spleen   F. Stomach
C. Vertebra   G. Descending aorta
D. Kidney

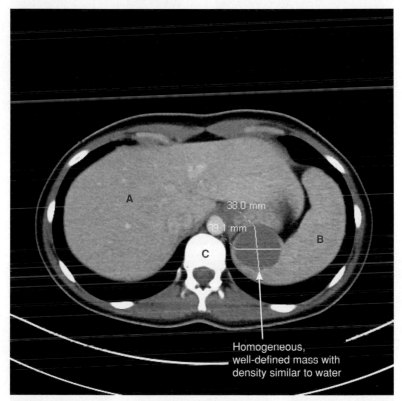

Homogeneous, well-defined mass with density similar to water

FIGURE 11.2 A

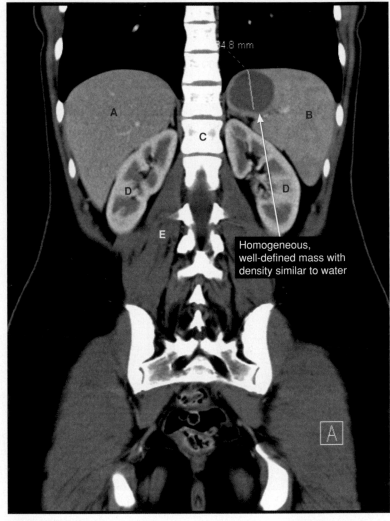

FIGURE 11.2 B

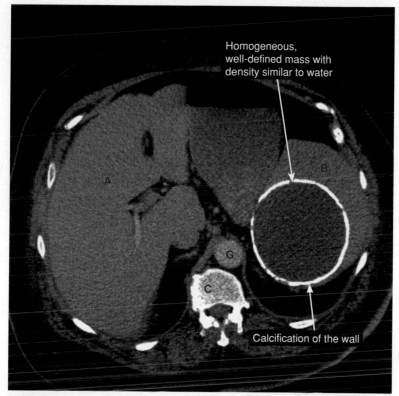

Homogeneous,
well-defined mass with
density similar to water

Calcification of the wall

FIGURE 11.2 C

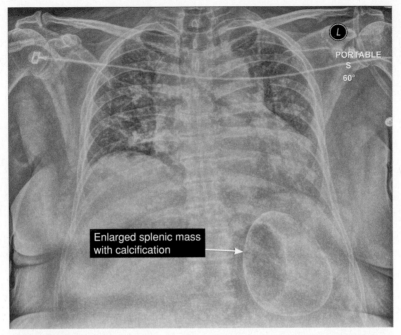

FIGURE 11.2 D

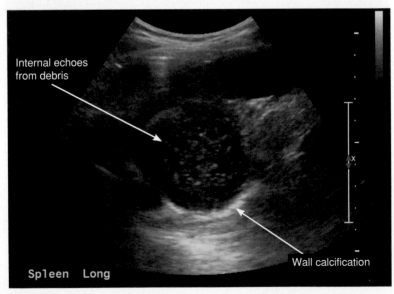

FIGURE 11.2 E

Splenic Infarction

Overview

- Multiple etiologies: Hypercoagulable state, embolic event, hematologic disorders (for example: sickle cell anemia etc.)
- Can also occur as a result of splenic vein thrombosis
- Infarct may be segmental or it may involve the entire spleen

Signs and Symptoms

- Abdominal pain (may or may not be left-sided), possible fever/ chills, nausea or vomiting, constitutional symptoms, elevated LDH, leukocytosis

Diagnosis

- CT scan is the preferred method

Treatment

- Observation, treat the underlying disorder, manage the patient's pain, close follow-up
- Only proceed with splenectomy if complications occur (for example: splenic rupture, splenic abscess, etc.), or variceal bleeding in the case of splenic vein thrombosis
- Administer vaccinations for encapsulated bacteria (*Streptococcus pneumoniae, Haemophilus influenzae, Neisseria meningitidis*) at the time of diagnosis in case patient may subsequently need to undergo splenectomy

RADIOLOGY

- **US findings**
  - Decreased echogenicity in a regional distribution
- **CT findings** (Fig. 11.3)
  - Well-defined areas of decreased attenuation are seen, usually wedge-shaped towards the periphery
- **MRI findings**
  - Wedge-shaped nonenhancing defects towards the periphery of the spleen which may be T1 hypointense and T2 hyperintense

FIGURE 11.3 A,B

A. Liver   D. Vertebra
B. Spleen   E. Descending aorta
C. Kidney

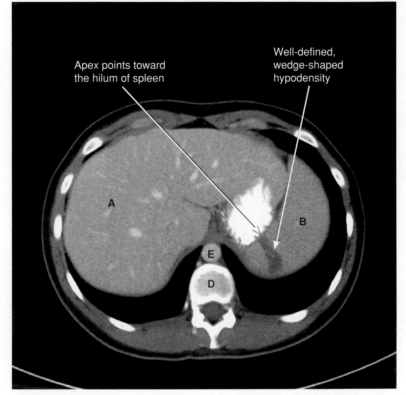

FIGURE 11.3 A

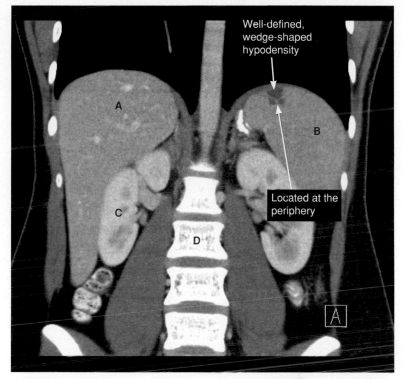

FIGURE 11.3 B

Splenomegaly

Overview

- Median weight for a spleen in adults is about 150 g
- Median size is about 8 to 11 cm, upper limit is <13 cm
- Splenomegaly defined as weight greater than 500 grams with the length greater than 15 cm
- Acts as a blood filter for red blood cells, platelets, bacteria
- Plays an important role in removing encapsulated bacteria (*Streptococcus pneumoniae, Haemophilus influenza, Neisseria meningitidis*)
- Etiologies of splenomegaly
  - Increased function: Spherocytosis, thalassemia, etc.
  - Infection: Mononucleosis, splenic abscess, etc.
  - Malignancy: Leukemia, lymphoma
  - Vascular: Thrombosis of the portal system, splenic vein thrombosis, etc.
  - Organ failure: Congestive heart failure, cirrhosis

RADIOLOGY

- **CT findings** (Fig. 11.4)
  - Spleen length of greater than 13 cm in the craniocaudal dimension

SWBH Library Services

City Hospital Library
Tel: 0121 507 5245

Borrowed Items 25/09/2014 17:16
XXX1215

Item Title	Due Date
* Imaging for surgical disease	23/10/2014
Breast Cancer	23/10/2014
Pathology	23/10/2014
Differential diagnosis	23/10/2014

* Indicates items borrowed today
Thank you for using this unit

FIGURE 11.4 A–C

A. Liver
B. Spleen
C. Stomach

D. Descending aorta
E. Vertebra
F. Gallbladder

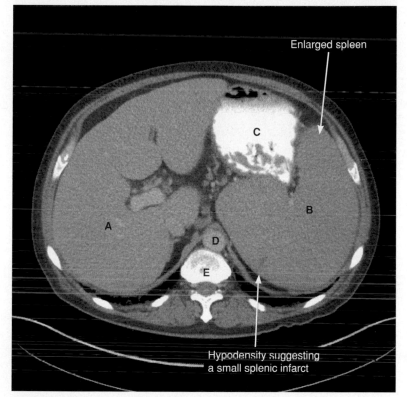

FIGURE 11.4 A

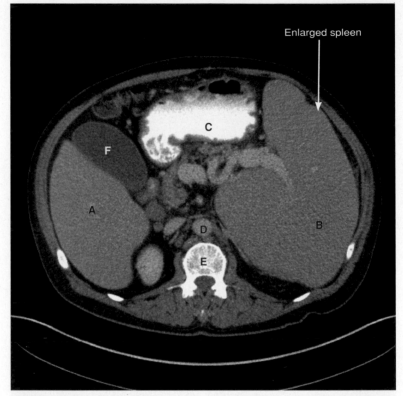

Enlarged spleen

FIGURE 11.4 B

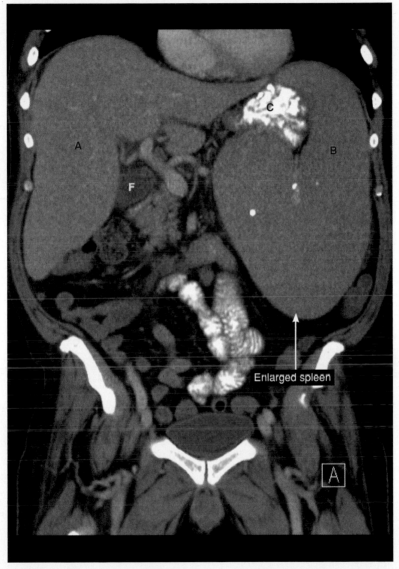

FIGURE 11.4 C

Suggested Readings

Agrawal GA, Johnson PT, Fishman EK. Splenic artery aneurysms and pseudoaneurysms: Clinical distinctions and CT appearances. *AJR Am J Roentgenol.* 2007;188:992–999.

Al-Habbal Y, Christophi C, Muralidharan V. Aneurysms of the splenic artery—a review. *Surgeon.* 2010;8(4):223–231.

Bezerra AS, D'Ippolito G, Faintuch S, et al. Determination of splenomegaly by CT: Is there a place for a single measurement? *AJR Am J Roentgenol.* 2005;184:1510–1513.

Lakin RO, Bena JF, Sarac TP, et al. The contemporary management of splenic artery aneurysms. *J Vasc Surg.* 2011;53(4):958–964.

Lawrence YR, Pokroy R, Berlowitz D, et al. Splenic infarction: An update on William Osler's observations. *Isr Med Assoc J.* 2010;12(6):362–365.

Morgenstern L. Nonparasitic splenic cysts: Pathogenesis, classification, and treatment. *J Am Coll Surg.* 2002;194(3):306–314.

Nores M, Phillips EH, Morgenstern L, et al. The clinical spectrum of splenic infarction. *Am Surg.* 1998;64(2):182–188.

Picardi M, Martinelli V, Ciancia R, et al. Measurement of spleen volume by ultrasound scanning in patients with thrombocytosis: A prospective study. *Blood.* 2002;99(11):4228–4230.

Sinha CK, Agrawal M. Nonparasitic splenic cysts in children: Current status. *Surgeon.* 2011;9(1):49–53.

Sprogoe-Jakobsen S, Sprogoe-Jakobsen U. The weight of the normal spleen. *Forensic Sci Int.* 1997;88(3):215–223.

Urrutia M, Mergo PJ, Ros LH, et al. Cystic masses of the spleen: Radiologic-pathologic correlation. *Radiographics.* 1996;16:107–129.

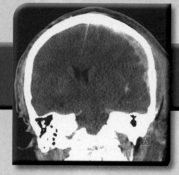

Trauma

Traumatic Brain Injury

Overview

Head CT indications in the trauma setting:

- GCS <15 two hours after injury or any GCS deterioration
- Suspected skull fractures
- Signs of basal skull fracture
- Loss of consciousness, persistent antegrade amnesia
- Dangerous mechanism (For example: ejection from motor vehicle)
- Elderly population age >60
- Drug or ETOH intoxication or inappropriate mental status
- Seizure or focal neurologic deficit
- Coagulopathy
- Trauma above the level of clavicle

Skull Fractures

- Described based upon the following characteristics:
  - Open vs. closed
  - Depressed vs. nondepressed
  - Linear vs. comminuted

Epidural Hematoma

- Hematoma between the dura and the skull
- Lateral fracture of skull resulting in disruption of middle meningeal artery or nearby vessel
- Convex appearance
- Presents as lucid interval: Temporary improvement in consciousness followed by deterioration

RADIOLOGY

- **CT findings** (Fig. 12.1)
  - Lentiform-shaped hyperdense area immediately deep to the skull, often in the temporal or parietal regions
  - Does not cross cranial sutures
  - Areas of hypodensity may indicate active hemorrhage

FIGURE 12.1

A. Epidural hematoma
B. Frontal lobe
C. Temporal lobe
D. Cerebellum
E. Pons
F. Petrous pyramid

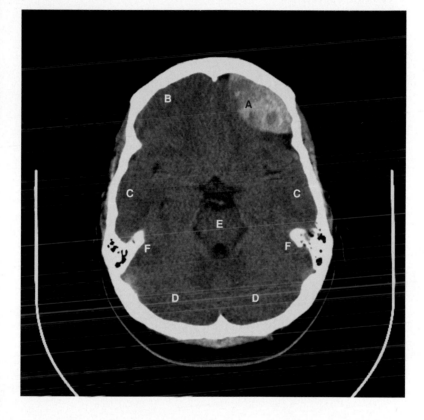

Subdural Hematoma

- Hematoma between the dura and the cortex
- Due to tearing of bridging veins
- Concave appearance

RADIOLOGY

Subdural Hematoma

- **CT findings** (Fig. 12.2)
  - Usually seen as hyperdense fluid layering over the cerebral convexities or along the falx cerebri which appears thickened
  - If acute, the blood will be hyperdense, but if chronic, the blood will be mixed in density
  - Blood decreases in density over time with a similar density to CSF after a few weeks to months

FIGURE 12.2 A–C

FIGURE 12.2 A

A. Subdural hematoma
B. Right-to-left midline shift
C. Lateral ventricles

D. Falx cerebri
E. Scalp hematoma

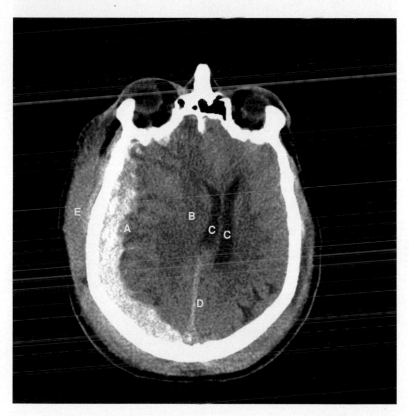

FIGURE 12.2 B

A. Subdural hematoma
B. Right-to-left midline shift
C. Lateral ventricles
D. Falx cerebri
E. Tentorium cerebelli
F. Cerebellum
G. Scalp hematoma

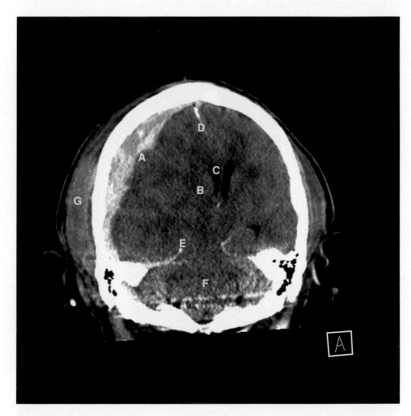

FIGURE 12.2 C

A. Subdural hematoma
B. Occipital lobe
C. Scalp hematoma
D. Tentorium cerebelli
E. Cerebellum

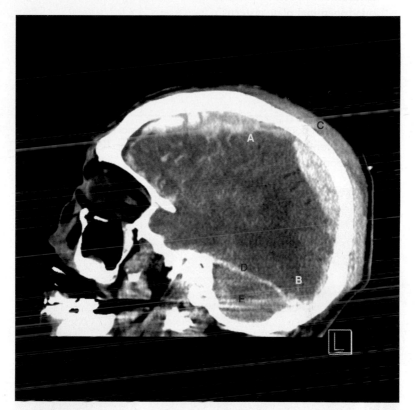

Subdural Hematoma with Diffuse Cerebral Edema

- ■ **CT findings** (Fig. 12.3)
  - • Effacement of cerebral sulci, as well as the suprasellar and quadrigeminal plate cisterns
  - • Compression of ventricular systems may be seen
  - • Edema causes diffuse decreased attenuation of the brain parenchyma with loss of the gray–white junction

FIGURE 12.3

A. Subdural hematoma
B. Narrowed ventricles from edema
C. Parietal bone fracture

D. Loss of sulci
E. Diffuse scalp hematoma

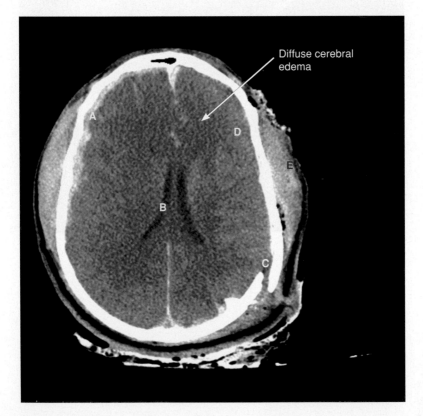

Diffuse cerebral edema

Subarachnoid Hemorrhage

- Bleeding into the subarachnoid space (area between the pia mater and the arachnoid membrane)
- Disruption of vessels feeding the cortex
- Signifies traumatic brain injury

RADIOLOGY

Subarachnoid Hemorrhage (SAH)

- **CT findings** (Fig. 12.4)
  - Hyperdense fluid that follows the sulci and gyri of the cerebrum (unlike subdural hemorrhages)
  - Blood within the ventricles, cisterns, and spinal canal can also be seen
- **MRI findings**
  - Dark, "blooming" artifact is seen with blood on T2* GRE
  - Failure to suppress the CSF on FLAIR sequences may indicate blood (which appears as bright fluid around the cerebral sulci and hyri)
  - If chronic SAH, a thin layer of T2 hypointense signal outlining the leptomeninges, especially in the basal cisterns can be seen

FIGURE 12.4 A–C
_____

FIGURE 12.4 A
_____

A. Subarachnoid hemorrhage
B. Falx cerebri
C. Lateral ventricles

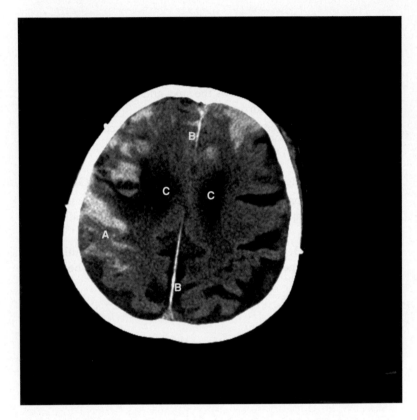

FIGURE 12.4 B

A. Subarachnoid hemorrhage
B. Falx cerebri
C. Anterior horn of lateral ventricles
D. Temporal horn of lateral ventricles
E. Third ventricle
F. Gyrus
G. Sulcus
H. Tentorium cerebelli
I. Pons

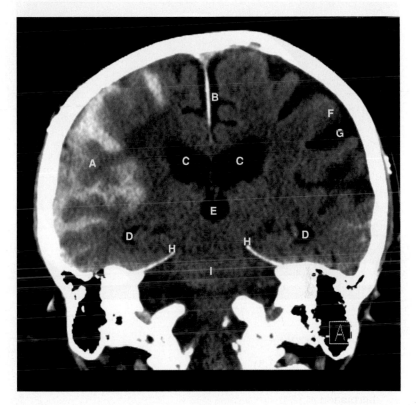

FIGURE 12.4 C

A. Subarachnoid hemorrhage
B. Lateral ventricle
C. Occipital lobe
D. Cerebellum

E. Pons
F. Parietal lobe
G. Pituitary

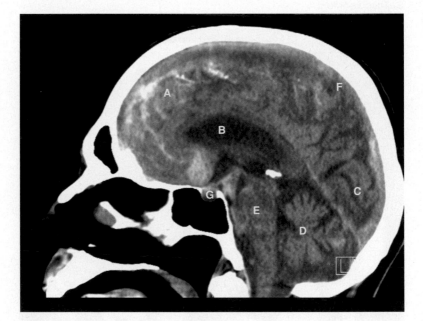

Brain Herniation

- **CT findings** (Fig. 12.5)
  - Subfalcine herniation is the most common form of brain herniation
  - Cingulate gyrus is displaced across the midline under the falx cerebri
  - Compression of adjacent lateral ventricle may be seen
  - Patients are at risk of anterior cerebral artery infarction in the distribution of the callosomarginal branch, where it is susceptible to compression against the falx cerebri

FIGURE 12.5 A–C

FIGURE 12.5 A

A. Subfalcine herniation
B. Left-to-right midline shift
C. Lateral ventricles

D. Posterior horn of lateral ventricles

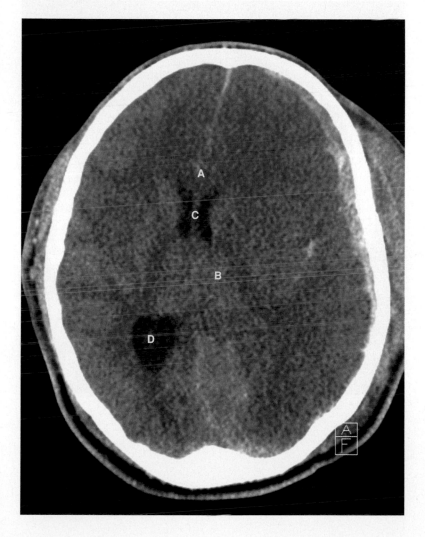

FIGURE 12.5 B

A. Subfalcine herniation
B. Subdural hematoma
C. Left-to-right midline shift
D. Lateral ventricles
E. Anterior horn of lateral ventricles
F. Subarachnoid hemorrhage

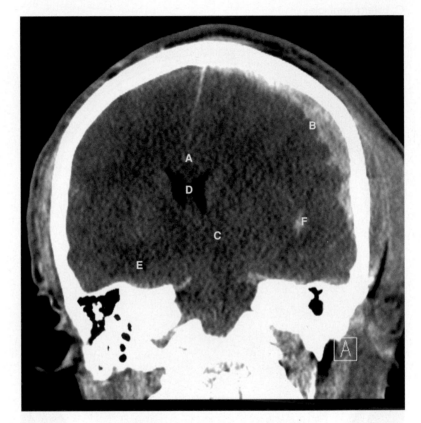

FIGURE 12.5 C

A. Tonsillar herniation
B. Transtentorial herniation
C. Cerebellum
D. Occipital lobe
E. Tentorium cerebelli
F. Lateral ventricle
G. Parietal lobe
H. Frontal lobe
I. Scalp hematoma

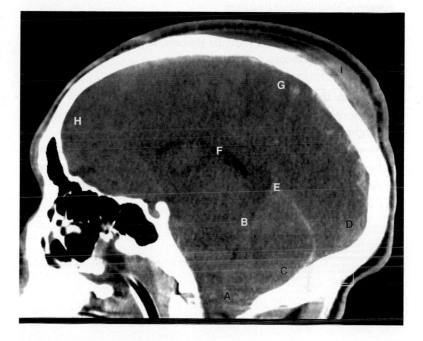

Intraparenchymal Hemorrhage

- Bleeding into the brain parenchyma
- Ranges from small contusions to large hematoma

Diffuse Axonal Injury

- Severe rotational forces lead to shear injury to white matter pathways
- Not directly seen on CT imaging but suggested by
  - punctate hemorrhages
  - loss of the gray/white matter differentiation

Spinal Injuries

Overview (Illustration 1)

- Anterior column: Anterior half of the vertebral body and disc, anterior longitudinal ligament
- Middle column: Posterior half of the vertebral body and disc, posterior longitudinal ligament
- Posterior column: Pedicles, lamina, ligamentum flavum, transverse process, spinous process, articular process, supraspinous and interspinous ligaments, joint capsules
- Instability:
  - Fracture that disrupts two of the three columns
  - Compression with reduction of more than 50% of vertebral height
  - More than 2.5 mm sagittal plane displacement of the vertebral body
  - Angulation of more than 20 degrees in the sagittal plane

ILLUSTRATION 1

Spine anatomy

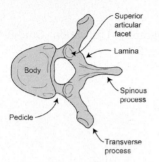

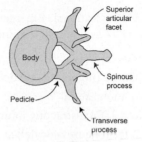

Thoracic Vertebra

Lumbar Vertebra

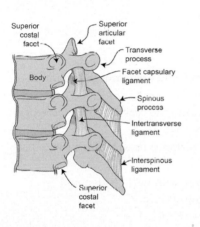

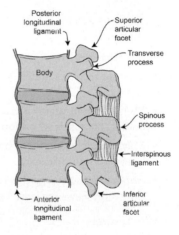

Cervical Spine Injuries (C-spine)

- One-third occur at level of C2
- One-half occur at level of C6–C7

NEXUS (National Emergency X-Radiography Utilization Study) criteria—C-spine is determined to be stable if:

C-spine injuries

- GCS 15 (no neurologic deficit)
- No intoxication
- No painful distracting injury
- No focal neurologic deficit
- No posterior midline tenderness

RADIOLOGY

- **Plain film findings**
  - Trauma series includes AP, lateral, and open mouth (odontoid views)
  - Malalignment of any element within the cervical spine (vertebral bodies, facet joints, spinous processes, etc.)
  - May see increased interspinous distance or widening of the intervertebral disc spaces
  - Abnormal motion of the vertebrae with neck flexion and extension views indicate ligamentous injury
- **CT findings**
  - More sensitive examination for cervical spine injuries (Fig 12.6 A-D)
  - Provides more detail of the extent of injury seen on plain film
- **MRI findings**
  - More sensitive examination for soft tissue injuries such as ligament tears
  - Examination of choice to evaluate for spinal cord injuries
  - Can detect epidural/subdural hematomas within the spinal canal

FIGURE 12.6 A–D

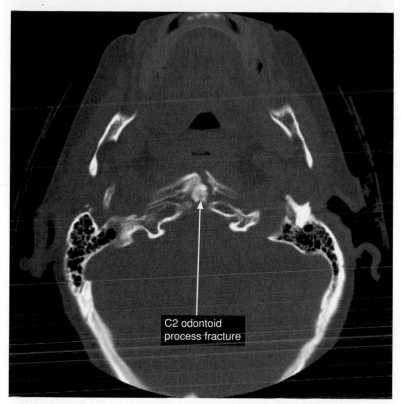

FIGURE 12.6 A

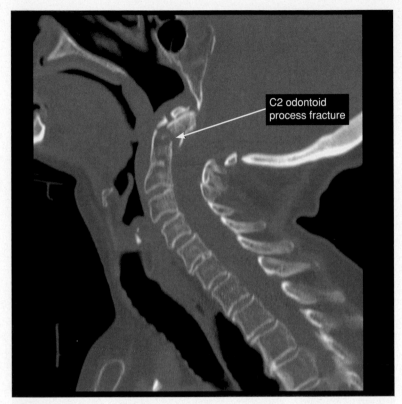

C2 odontoid process fracture

FIGURE 12.6 B

FIGURE 12.6 C

A. Vertebral body

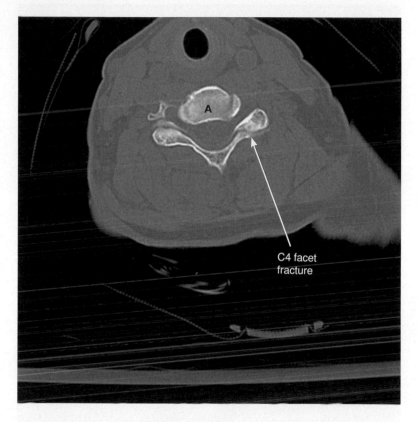

C4 facet
fracture

FIGURE 12.6 D

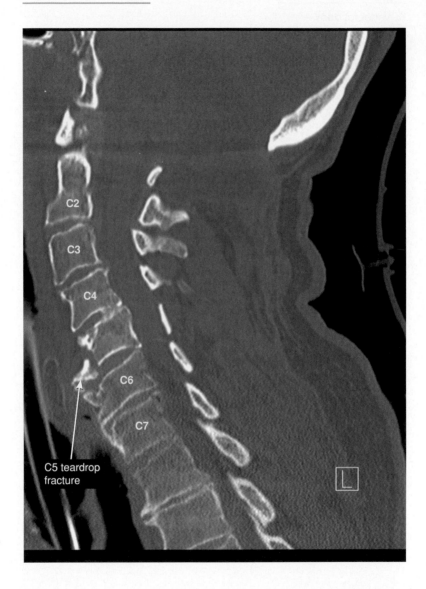

Flexion Injuries

- Simple wedge (Illustration 2)
  - Anterior body wedging
  - Decreased vertebral body height, increased density on imaging
  - Stable

ILLUSTRATION 2

Simple wedge fracture

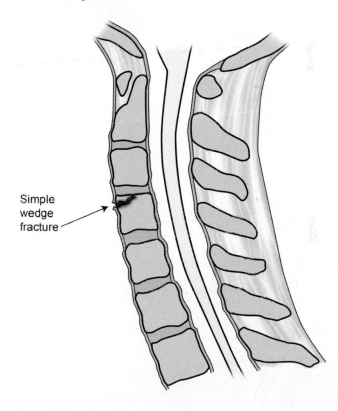

Simple wedge fracture

- Flexion teardrop (Illustration 3)
  - Flexion with vertical axial compression
  - Fracture of anteroinferior aspect of vertebral body with displacement
  - Involves disruption of all three columns and associated with cord injury
  - Unstable

ILLUSTRATION 3

Flexion teardrop

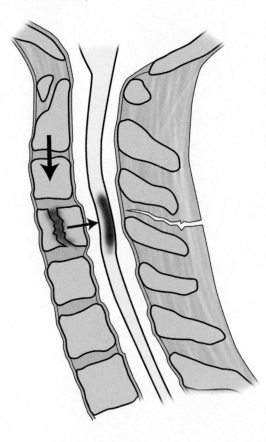

- Anterior subluxation (Illustration 4)
  - Rupture of posterior ligamentous structures
  - Widening of interspinous space seen on lateral view
  - Stable, but rarely associated with neurologic deficit, most are treated as unstable

ILLUSTRATION 4

Anterior subluxation

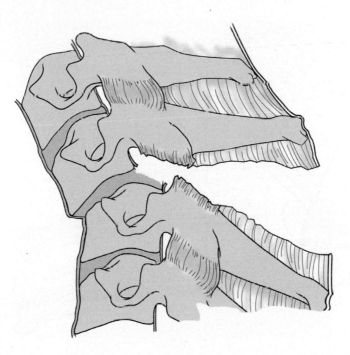

- Bilateral facet dislocation (Illustration 5)
  - Anterior subluxation with displacement of more than half of AP diameter, resulting in a "locked facet"
  - Associated with disk rupture
  - Unstable

ILLUSTRATION 5

Bilateral facet dislocation

"Locked facet"

Displacement greater than 50%

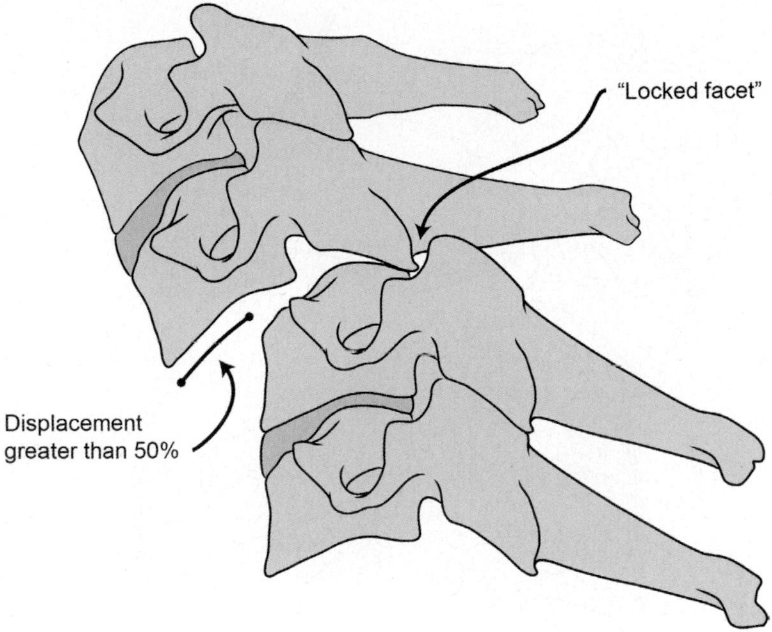

- Clay-shoveler (Illustration 6)
  - Abrupt flexion with neck contraction
  - Oblique fracture at base of spinous process, usually low C-spine
  - Stable

ILLUSTRATION 6

Clay shoveler

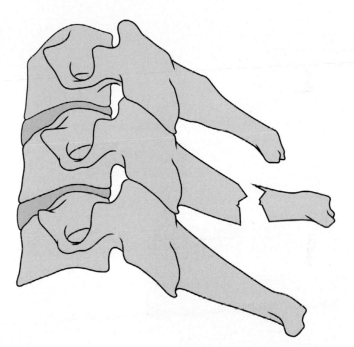

- Flexion–rotation (Illustration 7)
  - Unilateral facet dislocation
  - Inferior facet of upper vertebra passes superior and anterior to superior facet of lower vertebra
  - Disruption of posterior ligament
  - Anterior displacement < one-half of AP diameter of body on lateral view
  - Stable

Flexion–rotation

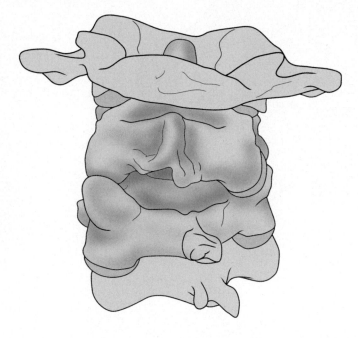

- Rotatory atlantoaxial dislocation (Illustration 8)
  - Specific unilateral facet dislocation
  - Asymmetry of C1 with respect to dens
  - Unstable

ILLUSTRATION 8

Rotatory atlantoaxial dislocation

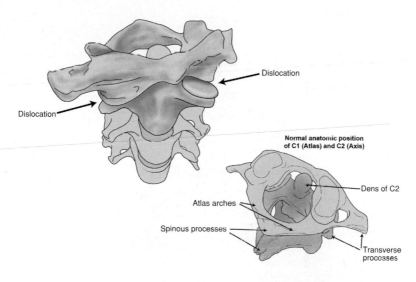

Dislocation

Dislocation

Normal anatomic position
of C1 (Atlas) and C2 (Axis)

Dens of C2

Atlas arches

Spinous processes

Transverse
processes

Extension Injuries

- Hangman fracture (Illustration 9)
  - Traumatic spondylolisthesis of C2
  - Bilateral fractures through pedicles of C2
  - Rarely associated with spinal cord injury
  - Unstable

ILLUSTRATION 9

Hangman fracture

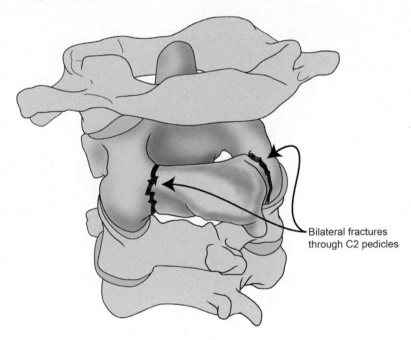

Bilateral fractures through C2 pedicles

- Extension teardrop (Illustration 10)
  - Anterior longitudinal ligament pulls away inferior aspect of vertebra
  - Hyperextension avulsion injury
  - Common in diving accidents
  - Unstable in extension (no traction)
  - Stable in flexion

ILLUSTRATION 10

Extension teardrop

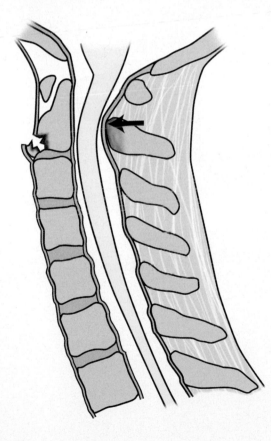

- Jefferson fracture (Illustration 11)
  - Burst fracture ring of C1
  - Fracture of anterior and posterior arches
  - Unstable

ILLUSTRATION 11

Jefferson fracture

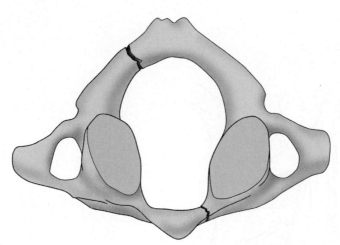

Thoracic and Lumbar Spine Injuries

RADIOLOGY

FIGURE 12.7 A,B

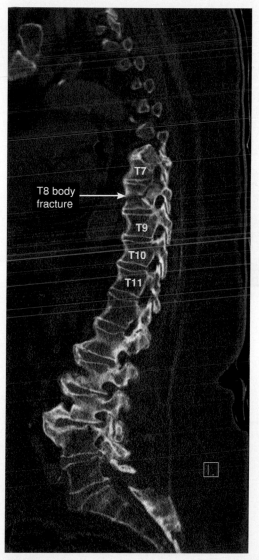

FIGURE 12.7 A

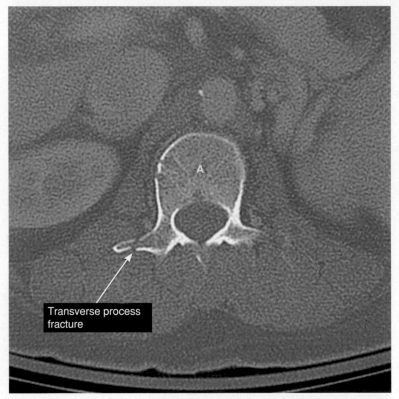

Transverse process
fracture

FIGURE 12.7 B

Flexion/Compression

- Wedge and compression fractures (Illustration 12)
  - Anterior column only—stable
  - Anterior and posterior column—potentially unstable
  - Three column—unstable with possible cord, nerve root, or vascular injury

ILLUSTRATION 12

Wedge and compression fracture

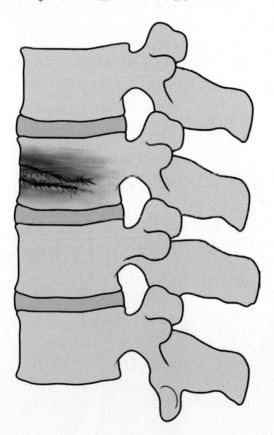

- Axial compression
  - Burst fracture (Illustration 13)
  - Anterior and middle columns compressed leading to loss of vertebral height
- Five subtypes:
  1. Fracture of both endplates
  2. Fracture of superior endplate (most common)
  3. Fracture of inferior endplate
  4. Burst rotation
  5. Burst lateral flexion fracture
- Stable burst fractures do not involve posterior column
- Unstable burst fractures involve posterior column
- Imaging required to evaluate canal impingement

ILLUSTRATION 13

Burst fracture

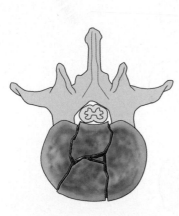
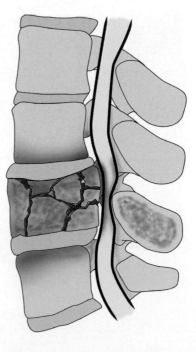

Flexion-Distraction

- Chance fracture (aka seatbelt injury) (Illustration 14)
  - Purely bony injury from posterior column to anterior column (spinous process, pedicles, and vertebral body)
  - Involves two to three columns of the spine, typically T10 to L2, any level may be affected

ILLUSTRATION 14

Chance fracture

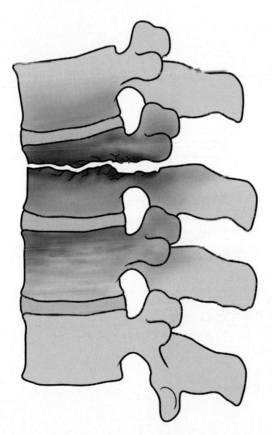

- Rotational fracture–dislocation (Illustration 15)
  - Lateral flexion and rotation
  - Middle and posterior column with varying degrees of anterior column involvement
  - Slice radiographic appearance
- Minor fractures
  - Transverse process, spinous process, pars interarticularis
  - All stable without neurologic involvement

ILLUSTRATION 15

Rotational fracture–dislocation

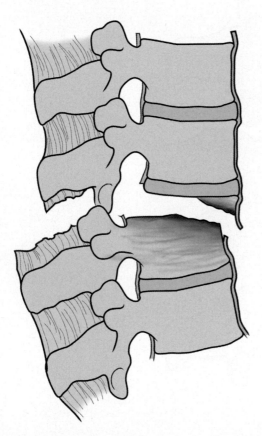

Thoracic Trauma

Etiology of Early Deaths

- Airway obstruction, flail chest, open pneumothorax, massive hemothorax, tension pneumothorax, cardiac tamponade

Hemothorax

- Blood within the pleural space
- Usually secondary to intercostal arterial bleeding
- May also be due to great vessels, lung parenchyma, or internal mammary injury
- Defined by size
  - Minimal <350 cc
  - Moderate 350 cc to 1500 cc
  - Massive >1500 cc
- 75% treated successfully with chest tube drainage alone
- 5% progress to empyema, 1% progress to fibrothorax
- Indications for thoracotomy
  - 1500 mL immediate output
  - 400 cc/h for 4 hours
  - 2 L within the first 24 hours
  - Esophageal or gastric contents noted

Pneumothorax

- Air in the pleural space
- Rupture or laceration of lung parenchyma
- 80% of traumatic pneumothoraces are associated with hemothorax
- Treatment: Tube thoracostomy
- An occult pneumothorax is seen on CT only and may possibly be treated with observation alone

Tension Pneumothorax

- Air is able to enter the pleural space without being able to escape (one way valve) leading to increased intrapleural pressure and causing a decrease in venous return
- Differentiated from simple pneumothorax by vital signs
- Tracheal/mediastinal shift *away* from tension pneumothorax
- Treatment: Needle thoracotomy followed by tube thoracostomy

RADIOLOGY

Diaphragmatic Injury with Pneumothorax

- **Plain film findings**
  - Hyperdense pleural line at the apex becomes separated from the chest wall by a zone devoid of vessels
  - Repeat radiograph taken with the patient in the decubitus position may clarify the pneumothorax if there is suspicion on the frontal radiograph
  - If patient is in the supine position, the following signs may be present:
    - Unilateral lucent lung
    - Deep costophrenic sulcus laterally (deep sulcus sign)
    - Focal lucency overlying the heart or lung, representing an anterior pneumothorax on a supine radiograph
    - Herniation of abdominal contents into the thorax
- **CT findings** (Fig. 12.8)
  - The underlying etiology such as a ruptured bleb can sometimes be seen in patients with a spontaneous pneumothorax
  - Disruption of the diaphragm is noted as protrusion of intra-abdominal organs into the thoracic cavity

FIGURE 12.8 A–C

FIGURE 12.8 A

A. Pneumothorax

B. Partially collapsed left lung

C. Subcutaneous emphysema

D. Right main bronchus

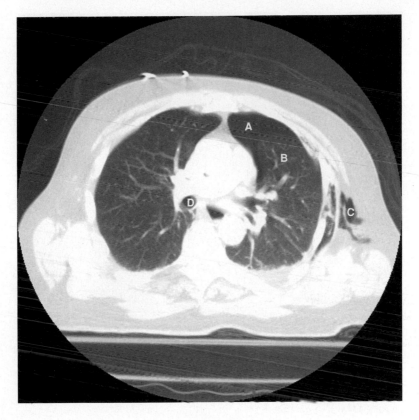

FIGURE 12.8 B,C

A. Liver
B. Portal vein
C. Right atrium
D. Left ventricle

E. Ascending aorta
F. Left atrium
G. Descending aorta
H. Vertebra

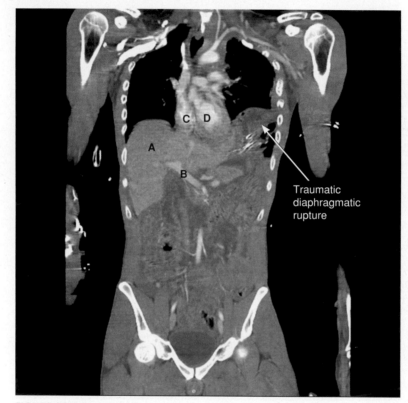

Traumatic
diaphragmatic
rupture

FIGURE 12.8 B

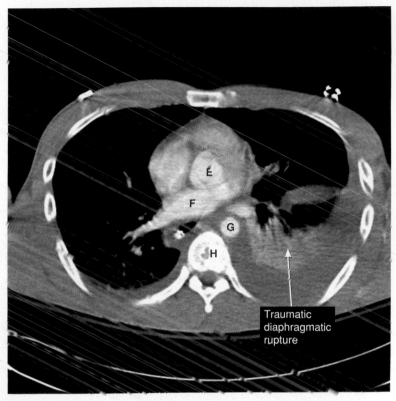

FIGURE 12.8 C

Chest Wall Trauma

- Most common thoracic injury associated with blunt trauma
- Associated with 100 cc blood loss/fracture
- Associated with hemothoraces, pulmonary contusions
- Treatment consists of adequate pain control
- Fractures of first to third ribs indicate severe trauma and other injuries such as vascular, brachial plexus, spinal, or tracheobronchial injuries should be suspected
- Fractures of tenth to twelfth ribs are associated with liver, spleen, or kidney injuries

Flail Chest

- An isolated segment of chest wall secondary to multiple rib fractures causing paradoxical movement
- Associated with underlying pulmonary contusion

RADIOLOGY

Rib Fracture

- **Plain film findings** (Fig. 12.9)
  - Rib fractures in children are uncommon
  - Due to the elasticity of the ribs in children, intrathoracic injuries such as aortic injury, tracheobronchial injury, or diaphragmatic rupture should be considered even if no rib fracture is present
  - Flail chest is defined as double fractures of three or more adjacent ribs
- **CT findings**
  - Much more sensitive in detecting more subtle, minimally displaced rib fractures

FIGURE 12.9

A. Bifurcation of trachea
B. Endotracheal tube
C. Fracture of right ribs 4–7

D. Fracture of left ribs 6–7
E. Subcutaneous emphysema
F. Dobhoff tube

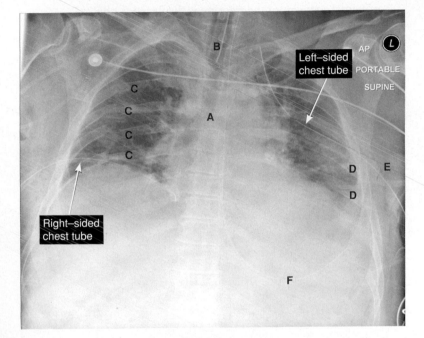

Clavicle Fracture

- **Plain film findings** (Fig. 12.10)
  - Can be either vertical or comminuted
  - Due to the superior pull of the sternocleidomastoid muscle, the proximal segment of the fracture is displaced cephalad

FIGURE 12.10

A. Left clavicle fracture
B. Left fifth rib fracture
C. Cardiac silhouette

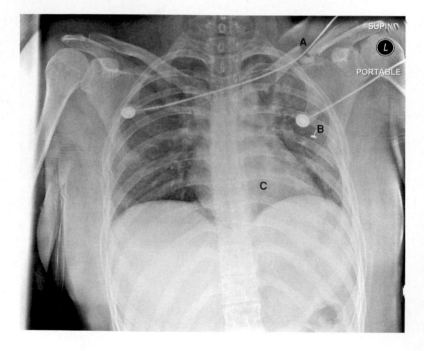

Chest Tube Placement

■ **Plain film findings** (Fig. 12.11)
- Chest tubes enter the lateral chest wall towards the mediastinum
- The sentinel hole, which allows communication with the pleural space, should be within the pleural space

FIGURE 12.11

A. Bifurcation of trachea
B. Endotracheal tube
C. Fracture of right ribs 4-7
D. Fracture of left ribs 6-7
E. Subcutaneous emphysema
F. Enteric tube

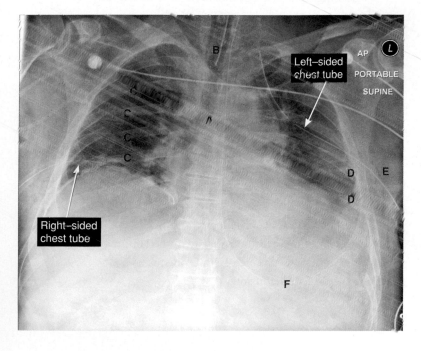

Pulmonary Contusion

- **Source of greatest physiologic insult**
  - Alveolar rupture with transudative fluid and blood extravasation causing localized airway obstruction and atelectasis
  - Leads to physiologic shunt with hypoxemia
  - Associated with strong inflammatory response
  - Usually associated with rib fractures
  - Radiographic findings usually progress (or become apparent) in 12 to 48 hours
  - Patchy parenchymal opacification/diffuse linear densities progressing to diffuse opacification (whited out lung)
  - May lead to pneumonia, ARDS

Vascular Injury

- Left-sided hematoma suggests descending aorta injury
- Right-sided hematoma suggests innominate injury
- >45% of patients with traumatic aortic injury surviving to ED injured just distal to left subclavian origin where aorta is tethered by the ligamentum arteriosum
- CXR findings suggesting aortic injury
  - Widened mediastinum
  - Blunting of the aortic knob
  - Tracheal or NG tube deviation
  - Left apical capping: Subtle opacity in the left lung apex
  - Depression of the left mainstem bronchus
  - Left-sided pleural effusion

Abdominal Trauma

- Diagnostic "black box"
- Nonoperative management in hemodynamically stable patients only
- Factors predicting failure of nonoperative management
  - High injury grade
  - Contrast extravasation on CT
  - Pseudoaneurysm
- Positive FAST and hemodynamic instability = exploratory laparotomy
- Positive FAST and hemodynamically stable = CT scan
  - CT indicated in stable patients without reliable examination
  - CT scan has limited ability to identify bowel injuries

Liver

- Involved in 2.9% of all traumas, 39.8% of all abdominal blunt trauma
- Frequently involved in upper abdominal penetrating trauma due to size
- Blunt trauma
  - Parenchyma and hepatic veins most likely injured
- Stab wounds
  - Linear tears
- Gunshot wounds
  - Cavitary injuries
- Indication for angiographic control
  - 4 units PRBC/6 hours without hemodynamic instability
  - 6 units PRBC/24 hours without hemodynamic instability
  - Rebleed within 24 to 48 hours
- Surgical options
  - Packing, local pressure, Pringle maneuver (does not stop hepatic vein bleeding), topical hemostasis

Solid Organ Injury Scale

Liver

Grade	Type	Description
I	Hematoma	Subcapsular <10% surface area
	Laceration	Capsular tear <1 cm depth
II	Hematoma	Subcapsular 10–50% surface area; intraparenchymal <10 cm in diameter
	Laceration	Capsular tear 1–3 cm in depth and <10 cm in length
III	Hematoma	Subcapsular 50% surface area; intraparenchymal >10 cm in diameter
	Laceration	>3 cm in depth
IV	Laceration	Parenchymal disruption involving 25–75% of hepatic lobe or 1 to 3 Couinaud segments within a single lobe
V	Laceration	Parenchymal disruption involving >75% of hepatic lobe or >3 Couinaud segments within a single lobe
	Vascular	Juxta-hepatic venous injuries
VI	Vascular	Hepatic avulsion

RADIOLOGY

- **CT findings** (Figs. 12.12–12.16)
  - CT-based injury severity of blunt hepatic trauma is classified into five grades

Grade I—Capsular avulsion, superficial laceration <1 cm deep, subcapsular hematoma <1 cm in maximum thickness, periportal blood tracking only

FIGURE 12.12 A,B

A. Stomach   D. Descending aorta
B. Kidneys   E. Portal vein
C. Spleen   F. Gallbladder

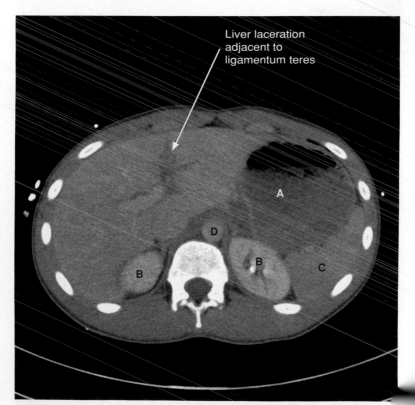

Liver laceration adjacent to ligamentum teres

FIGURE 12.12 A

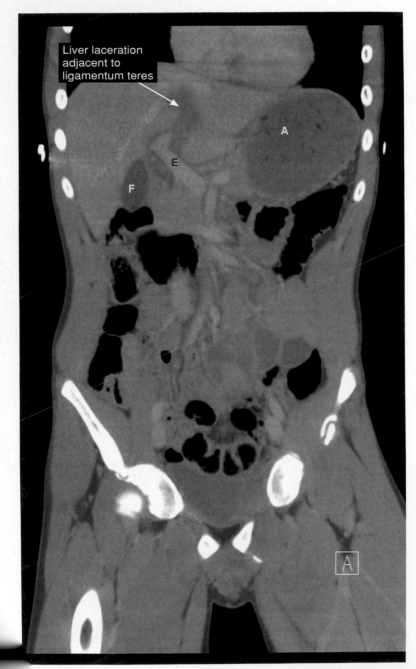

Liver laceration adjacent to ligamentum teres

Grade II—Laceration 1 to 3 cm deep, central-subcapsular hematoma 1 to 3 cm in diameter

FIGURE 12.13 A–C

A. Stomach
B. Kidneys
C. Spleen
D. Descending aorta

E. IVC
F. Gallbladder
G. Portal vein

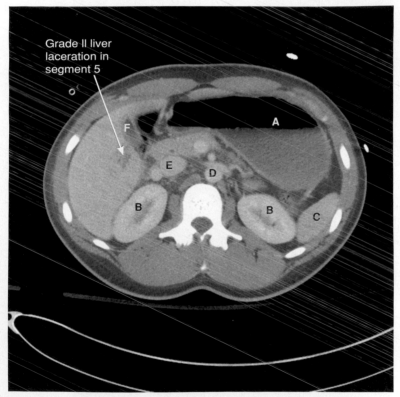

Grade II liver laceration in segment 5

FIGURE 12.13 A

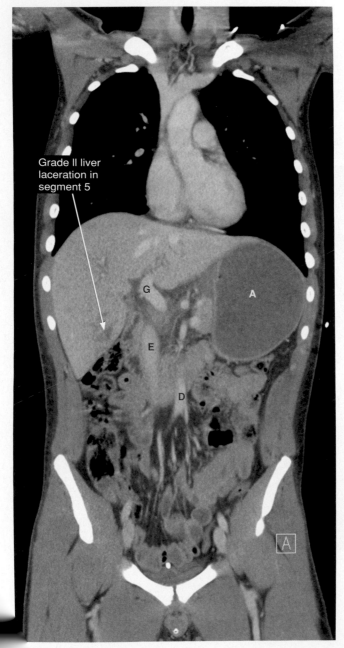

Grade II liver laceration in segment 5

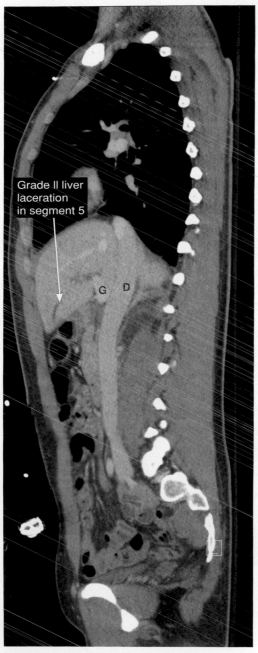

Grade II liver laceration in segment 5

G D

FIGURE 12.13 C

Grade III—Laceration greater than 3 cm deep, central-subcapsular hematoma >3 cm in diameter

FIGURE 12.14 A–C

A. Portal vein
B. IVC
C. Descending aorta
D. Vertebra
E. Stomach

F. Spleen
G. Small bowel loops
H. Kidney
I. Gallbladder

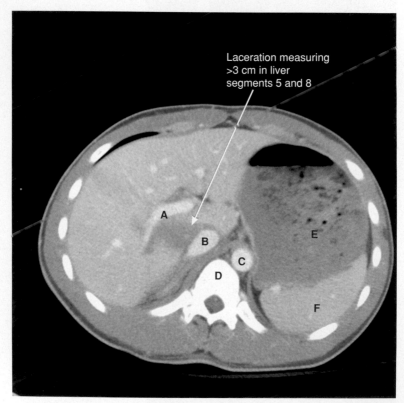

FIGURE 12.14 A

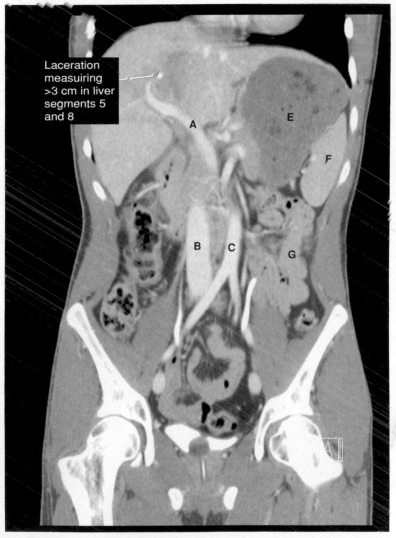

Laceration measuiring >3 cm in liver segments 5 and 8

FIGURE 12.14 B

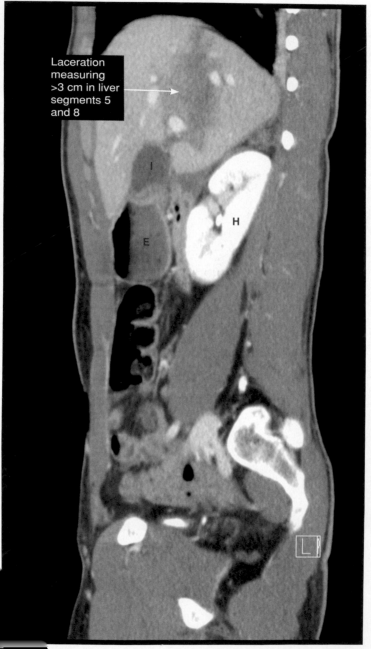

Laceration measuring >3 cm in liver segments 5 and 8

Grade IV—Massive central-subcapsular hematoma >10 cm, lobar
tissue destruction or devascularization

FIGURE 12.15 A–C

A. Stomach	E. Descending aorta
B. Spleen	F. Vertebra
C. Portal vein	G. Kidney
D. IVC	H. Fluid collection in Morrison's pouch

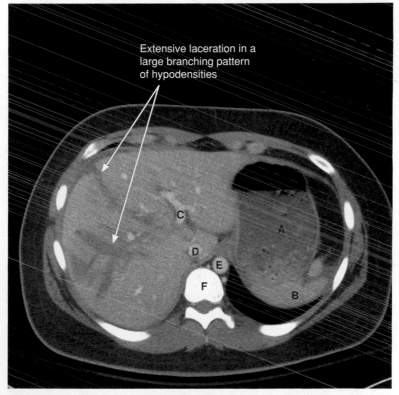

FIGURE 12.15 A

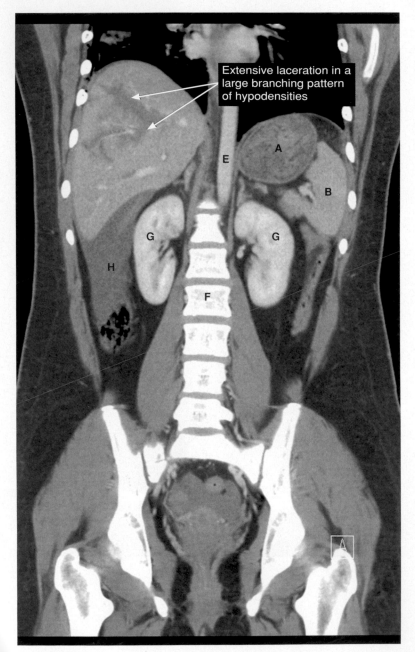

Extensive laceration in a large branching pattern of hypodensities

FIGURE 12.15 B

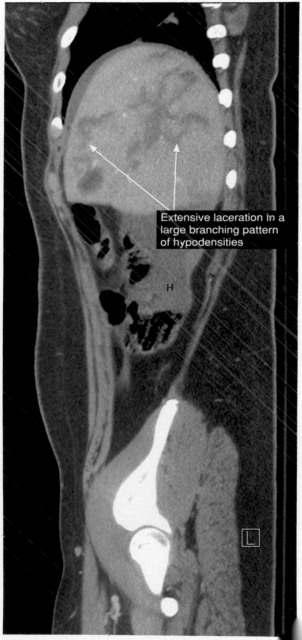

Extensive laceration in a large branching pattern of hypodensities

H

L

FIGURE 12.15 C

Grade V—Bilobar tissue destruction or devascularization

FIGURE 12.16 A,B

A. Gallbladder   E. IVC
B. Stomach   F. Descending aorta
C. Spleen   G. Vertebra
D. Portal vein   H. Perisplenic hematoma

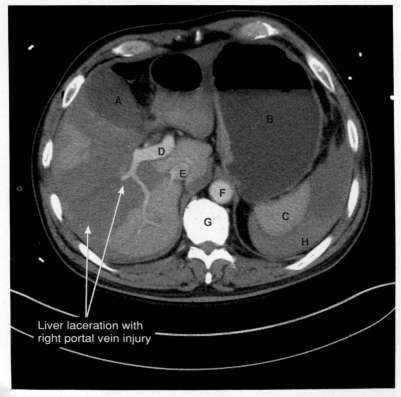

Liver laceration with right portal vein injury

FIGURE 12.16 A

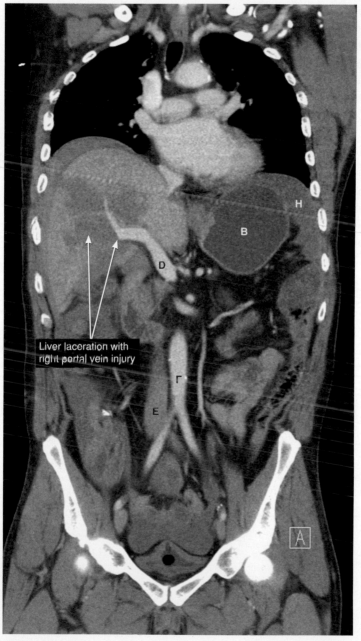

Liver laceration with right portal vein injury

FIGURE 12.16 B

Spleen

- Involved in 3.2% all trauma, 50% blunt abdominal trauma
- Most commonly injured abdominal organ in blunt trauma
- Injury from compression in left upper quadrant or deceleration (tearing capsule at fixed points)
- Best evaluated on CT in portal venous phase
- One-third of grade IV and three-fourth of grade V splenic injuries fail nonoperative management
- May rebleed weeks after injury
- Postsplenectomy vaccines
  - *Streptococcus pneumoniae, Neisseria meningitidis, Haemophilus influenza*

Grade	Injury	Description
I	Hematoma	Subcapsular <10% surface area
	Laceration	Capsular tear <1 cm depth
II	Hematoma	Subcapsular involving 10–50% surface area, intraparenchymal <5 cm in diameter
	Laceration	Capsular tear 1–3 cm in depth not involving trabecular vessel
III	Hematoma	Subcapsular >50% surface or expanding Ruptured subcapsular/parenchymal hematoma Intraparenchymal >5 cm or expanding
IV	Laceration	Involvement of segmental/hilar vessels with >25% devascularization
V	Hematoma	Shattered
	Laceration	Devascularized spleen from hilar vascular injury

RADIOLOGY

- **US findings**
  - Lacerations are typically hypoechoic regions, sometimes associated with perisplenic fluid
- **CT findings** (Figs. 12.17–12.20)
  - Linear, hypoattenuating region of the spleen on non-contrast images
  - Intraparenchymal hematoma may manifest as a hypodense area of nonperfused spleen on contrast-enhanced images
  - Subcapsular hematoma is seen as a crescentic fluid collection that distorts the underlying spleen
  - Perisplenic hematoma may be multilayered if multiple episodes of bleeding is present
  - Splenic injury scale according to AAST

Grade I—Subcapsular hematoma <10% surface area, capsular tear <1 cm parenchymal depth

FIGURE 12.17 A-C

FIGURE 12.17 A

A. Grade I splenic laceration with trace perisplenic fluid
B. Liver
C. Left kidney
D. Stomach
E. Descending aorta

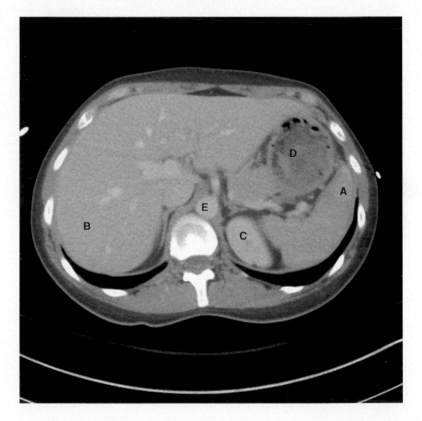

FIGURE 12.17 B

A. Grade I splenic laceration D. Psoas muscle
B. Liver   E. Stomach
C. Right kidney   F. Descending aorta

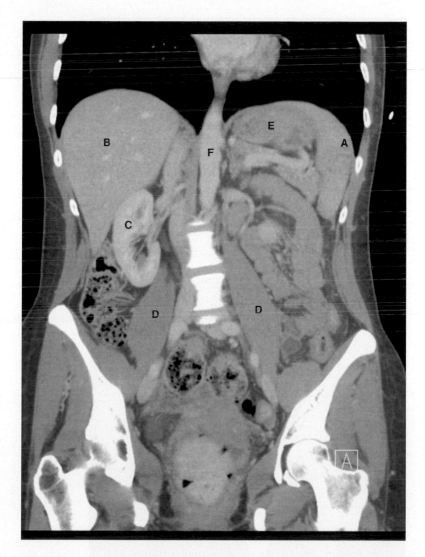

FIGURE 12.17 C

A. Grade I splenic laceration
B. Stomach
C. Small bowel loops

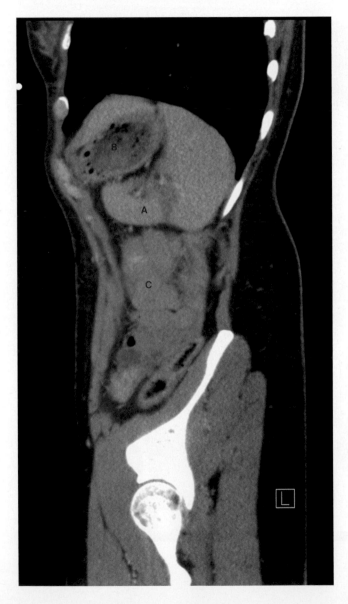

Grade II—Subcapsular hematoma 10% to 50% surface area, intraparenchymal hematoma <5 cm in diameter, laceration 1 to 3 cm parenchymal depth and does not involve a trabecular vessel

FIGURE 12.18 A,B

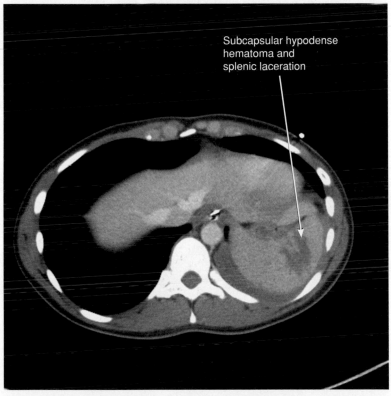

Subcapsular hypodense hematoma and splenic laceration

FIGURE 12.18 A

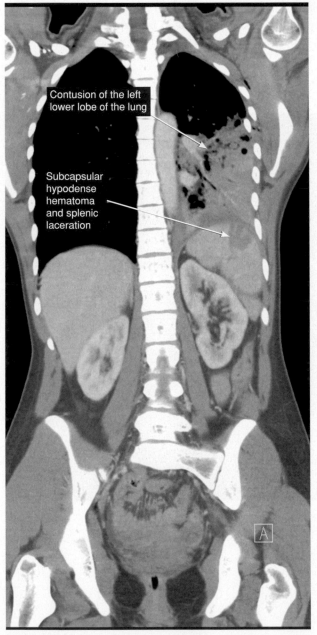

Contusion of the left lower lobe of the lung

Subcapsular hypodense hematoma and splenic laceration

FIGURE 12.18 B

Grade III—Subcapsular hematoma >50% surface area or expanding, ruptured subcapsular or parenchymal hematoma, laceration >3 cm parenchymal depth or involving trabecular vessels

FIGURE 12.19 A,B

FIGURE 12.19 A

A. Grade III splenic injury with surrounding hematoma

B. Liver with free fluid anteriorly

C. Stomach

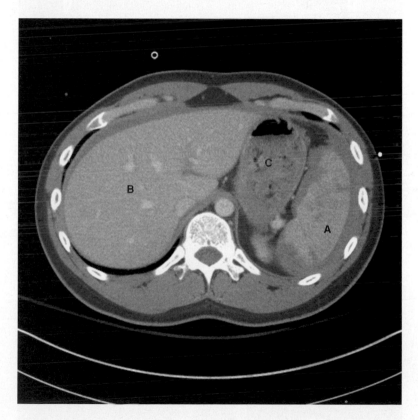

FIGURE 12.19 B

A. Grade III splenic injury with surrounding hematoma

B. Liver

C. Stomach

D. Small bowel loops

E. Psoas muscle

F. Descending aorta

G. Portal vein

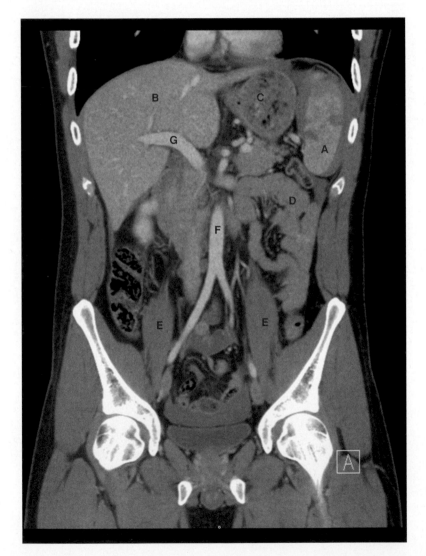

Grade IV—Laceration involving segmental or hilar vessels and producing major devascularization (>25% of spleen)

FIGURE 12.20 A,B

FIGURE 12.20 A

A. Grade IV splenic laceration with surrounding hematoma

B. Liver

C. Stomach

D. Descending aorta

E. Kidneys

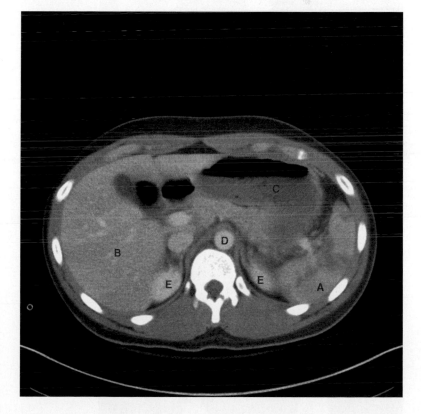

FIGURE 12.20 B

A. Grade IV splenic laceration with surrounding hematoma
B. Liver
C. Stomach
D. Kidneys
E. Psoas muscle
F. Colon
G. Descending aorta

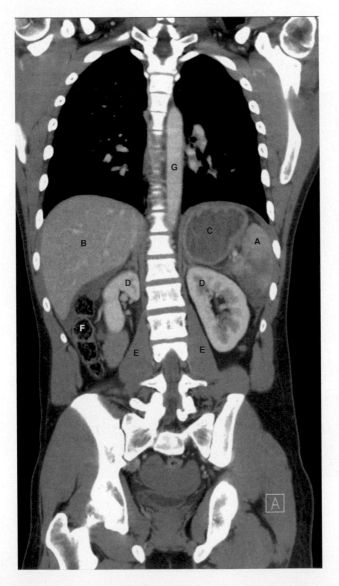

Kidney

- If suspicious of ureteral injury, evaluate with CT urogram

Grade	Injury	Description
I	Contusion	Micro/gross hematuria with normal imaging
	Hematoma	Subcapsular, nonexpanding, no parenchymal laceration
II	Hematoma	Nonexpanding perirenal hematoma, confined to renal retroperitoneum
	Laceration	<1 cm depth, no urine extravasation
III	Laceration	>1 cm depth without involvement of collection system, no urine extravasation
IV	Laceration	Parenchymal laceration through renal cortex, medulla, and collecting system
	Vascular	Main renal artery or vein injury with contained hemorrhage
V	Laceration	Shattered kidney
	Vascular	Avulsed hilum with devascularized kidney

RADIOLOGY

- **CT findings** (Figs. 12.21–12.25)
  - Renal injury is classified into five grades according to AAST
  - Important to obtain 10 minute delayed images if renal collecting system injury is suspected at the scanner to evaluate for a urinary leak

Grade I—Hematuria with normal imaging studies, renal contusion, nonexpanding subcapsular hematoma without parenchymal laceration

FIGURE 12.21 A,B

A. Kidney
B. Vertebra
C. Liver
D. Descending aorta

E. Small bowel loop
F. Splenic laceration and perisplenic hematoma
G. Psoas muscle

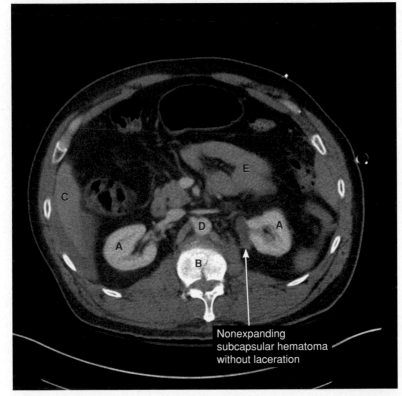

Nonexpanding subcapsular hematoma without laceration

FIGURE 12.21 A

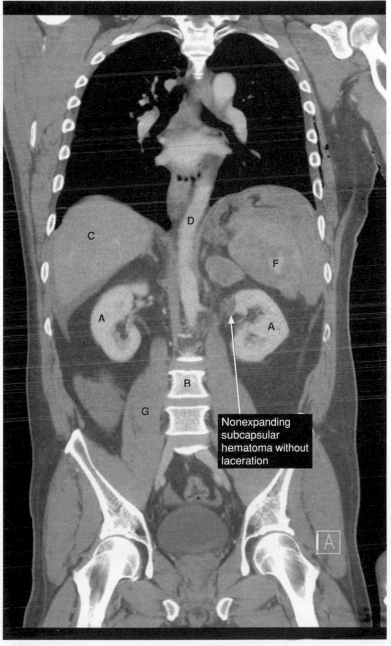

Nonexpanding subcapsular hematoma without laceration

FIGURE 12.21 B

Grade II—Nonexpanding perirenal hematoma confined to the retro-peritoneum, superficial lacerations <1 cm depth in the renal cortex

FIGURE 12.22 A–C

A. Liver
B. Kidney
C. Vertebra
D. Gallbladder
E. Small bowel loops
F. Spleen
G. Psoas muscle
H. Bladder
I. IVC
J. Abdominal aorta

Laceration measuring <1 cm in the anterior cortex

FIGURE 12.22 A

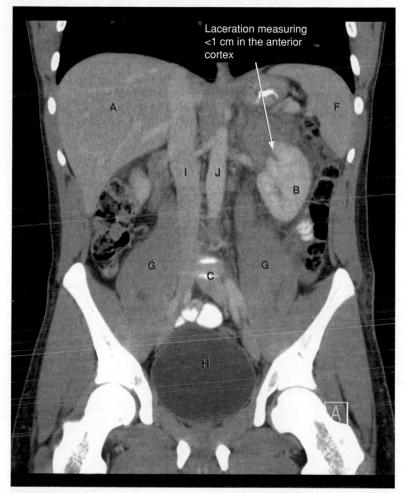

Laceration measuring
<1 cm in the anterior
cortex

FIGURE 12.22 B

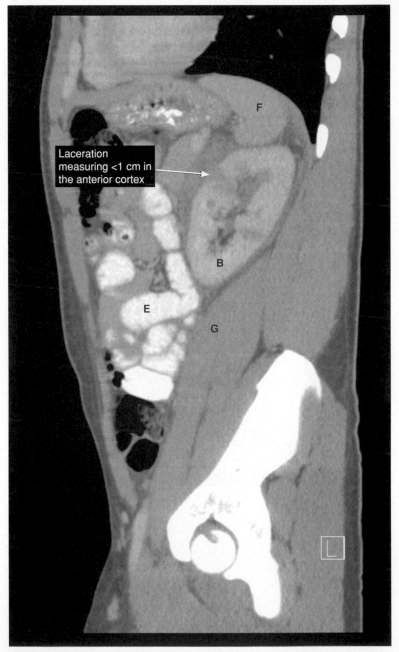

Laceration measuring <1 cm in the anterior cortex

F

B

E

G

L

FIGURE 12.22 C

Grade III—Lacerations >1 cm depth in the renal cortex without
extension into the collecting system or urinary extravasation

FIGURE 12.23 A–C

A. Liver   E. Spleen
B. Kidney   F. Psoas muscle
C. Vertebra   G. Small bowel loops
D. Stomach

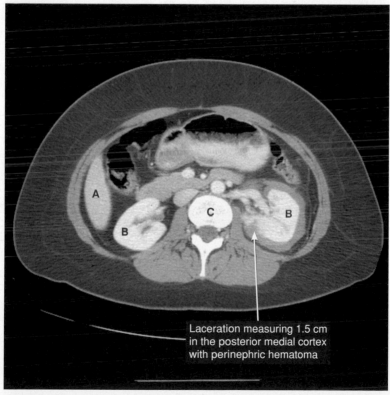

Laceration measuring 1.5 cm
in the posterior medial cortex
with perinephric hematoma

FIGURE 12.23 A

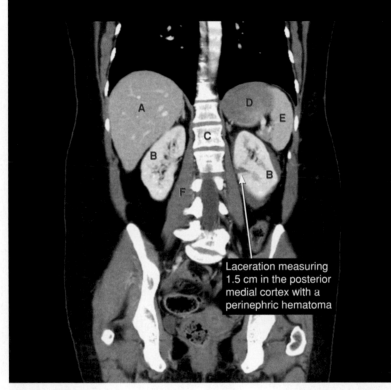

Laceration measuring 1.5 cm in the posterior medial cortex with a perinephric hematoma

FIGURE 12.23 B

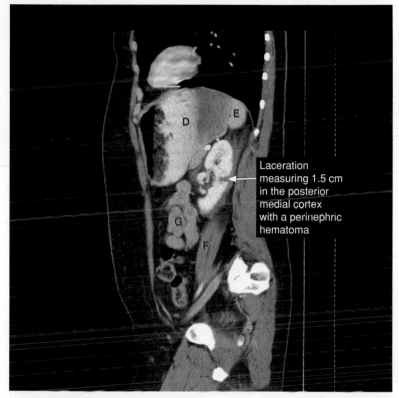

Laceration measuring 1.5 cm in the posterior medial cortex with a perinephric hematoma

FIGURE 12.23 C

Grade IV—Lacerations extending through the renal cortex, medulla, and collecting system; injuries to the main renal artery or vein with contained hemorrhage; thrombosis of a segmental renal artery without parenchymal laceration

FIGURE 12.24 A–C

A. Kidney

B. Vertebra

C. Small bowel loops

D. Liver

E. Spleen

F. Psoas muscle

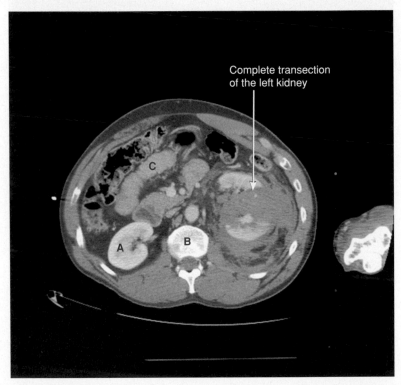

Complete transection of the left kidney

FIGURE 12.24 A

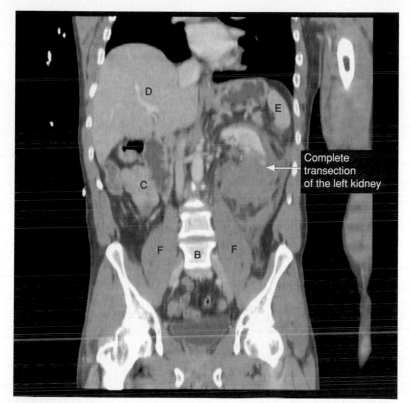

Complete transection of the left kidney

FIGURE 12.24 B

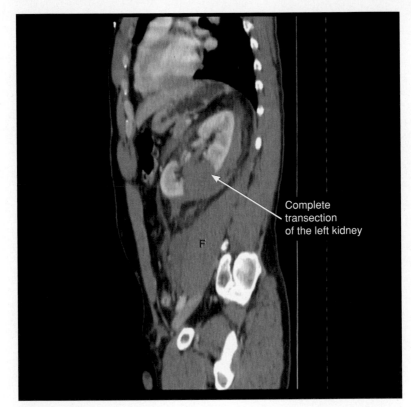

Complete
transection
of the left kidney

FIGURE 12.24 C

Grade V—Lacerations that completely shatter the kidney; injuries to the renal hilum with devascularization of the kidney: Traumatic renal arterial disruption and traumatic renal arterial occlusion

FIGURE 12.25 A–C

A. Liver
B. Gallbladder
C. Kidney
D. Vertebra
E. Stomach
F. Psoas muscle

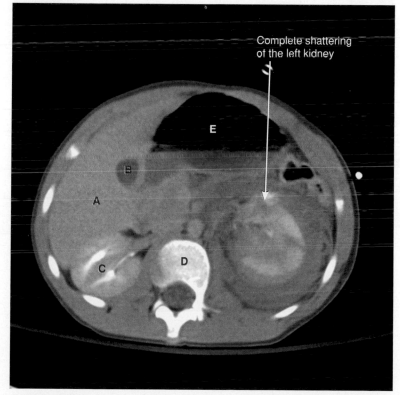

FIGURE 12.25 A

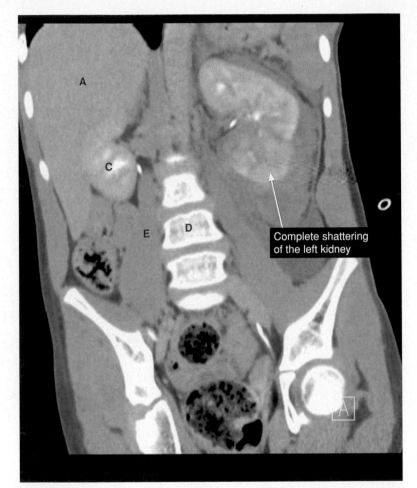

Complete shattering of the left kidney

FIGURE 12.25 B

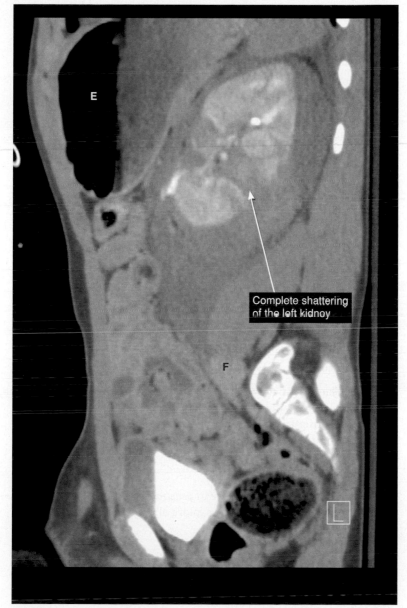

Complete shattering of the left kidney

FIGURE 12.25 C

Other Intra-abdominal Injuries

Duodenum

- Rarely injured (6% penetrating, 0.1% blunt)
- Blunt injury usually secondary to narrow epigastric strike
- Duodenal hematoma seen with IV contrast administration
  - Manage conservatively with NG tube, NPO, TPN
  - May have concurrent pancreatic injury
- If there is contrast extravasation
  - OR exploration

Pancreas

- If no ductal injury, may be observed
- If presence of ductal injury, OR exploration
- Diagnose ductal injury by performing ERCP or MRCP

Retroperitoneal Hematoma

Zone 1 (extends from the diaphragm to the area just distal to the bifurcation of aorta—aorta, IVC, duodenum, pancreas, renal pedicle)
Management: OR exploration

Zone 2 (lateral aspect of superior abdomen—kidney, adrenal, ureters, hilum of kidney)
Management: Only explore in *penetrating* injury, only explore in blunt injury if *expanding/pulsatile* hematoma or if there is extravasation of urine

Zone 3 (pelvic retroperitoneum)
Management: Only explore in *penetrating* injury.
That is, penetrating injury—explore all zones!! Blunt injury, only zone 1, ± zone 2 only

Bladder

- Diagnose with CT cystogram vs. fluorographic imaging
- **Intraperitoneal rupture**
  - A result of sudden compression to lower abdominal wall
  - Typically in the bladder dome
  - **Management:** OR exploration

■ **Extraperitoneal rupture**
  • More common
  • Lower bladder segment/anterolateral retropubic portion of bladder
  • Associated with pelvic fractures
  • **Management:** Nonoperatively with Foley catheter drainage

RADIOLOGY

Bladder Rupture

■ **Cystography findings**
  • Should be performed after ruling out urethral injury and when bladder catheterization is safe
  • Scout full bladder, and post void pelvic radiographs are obtained
  • Intraperitoneal bladder rupture usually occurs at the bladder dome
  • Most extraperitoneal bladder injuries occur in the anterolateral wall near the bladder base
  • In extraperitoneal bladder rupture, contrast is seen dissecting through fascial places and into the anterior prevesical space of Retzius, anterior abdominal wall, inguinal regions, lateral paravesical space, and presacral space
  • Contrast can also extend into the perineum and scrotum if there is disruption of the urogenital diaphragm and bladder base
  • Filling defects within the bladder may represent blood clots in the setting of trauma and can block a urine leak
■ **Plain film findings**
  • Cystography should be performed in patients with gross hematuria and pelvic fractures

- **CT findings** (Figs. 12.26, 12.27)
  - Usually performed with the injection of contrast into the bladder if the patient is admitted for trauma
  - More accurate than standard cystography for the detection of bladder injuries
  - Free contrast-enhanced urine pooling in the paravesical space causes a "molar tooth" appearance, indicating extraperitoneal bladder rupture

FIGURE 12.26 A,B

A. Air within small bowel loop	F. Bladder
B. Uterus	G. Iliac crest
C. Ilium	H. Pubis
D. Sacrum	I. Small bowel loops
E. Iliopsoas	

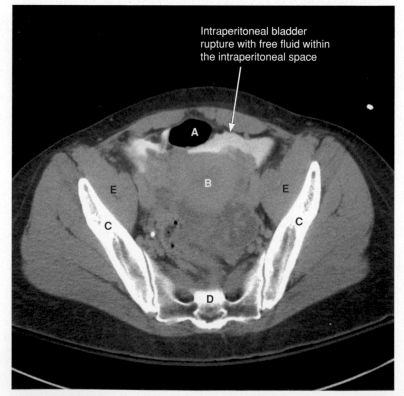

Intraperitoneal bladder rupture with free fluid within the intraperitoneal space

FIGURE 12.26 A

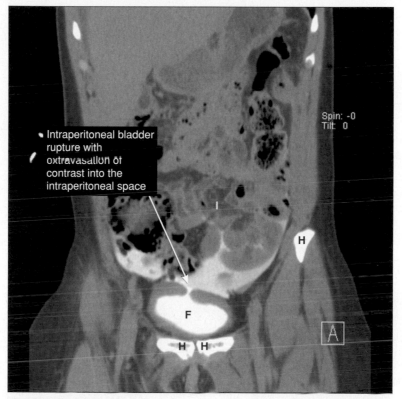

Intraperitoneal bladder rupture with extravasation of contrast into the intraperitoneal space

Spin: -0
Tilt: 0

FIGURE 12.26 B

Extraperitoneal Bladder Rupture

FIGURE 12.27 A–E

A. Bladder
B. Pubic symphysis
C. Sacrum
D. Ilium
E. Foley catheter in bladder

F. Head of femur
G. Anterior acetabulum
H. Posterior acetabulum
I. Rectum

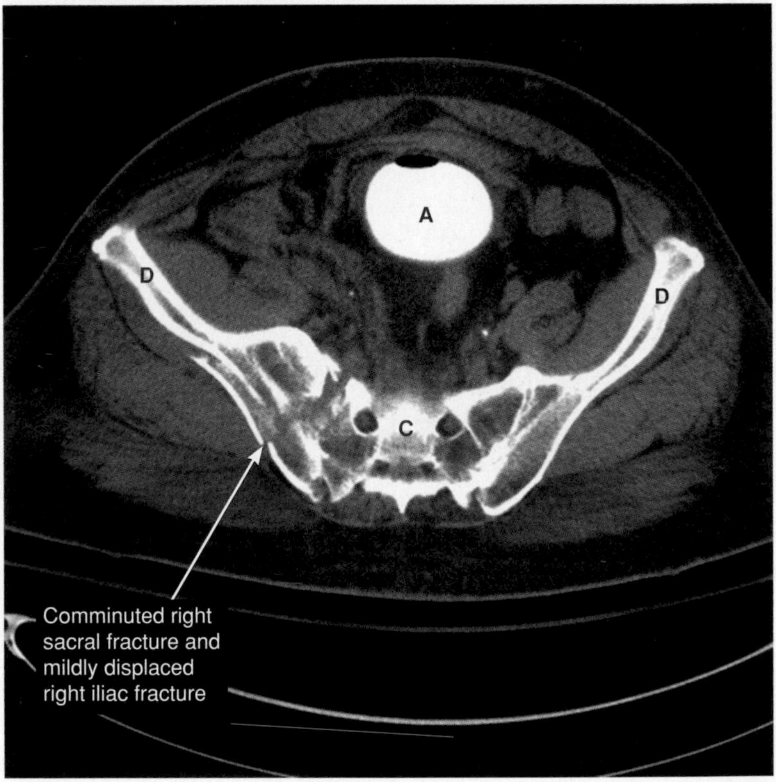

Comminuted right sacral fracture and mildly displaced right iliac fracture

FIGURE 12.27 A

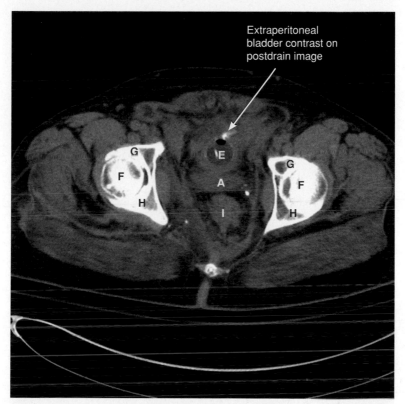

Extraperitoneal
bladder contrast on
postdrain image

FIGURE 12.27 B

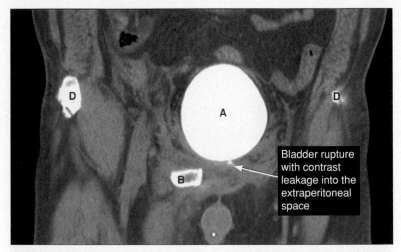

Bladder rupture with contrast leakage into the extraperitoneal space

FIGURE 12.27 C

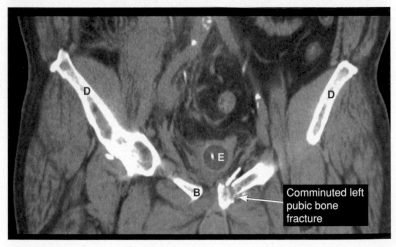

Comminuted left pubic bone fracture

FIGURE 12.27 D

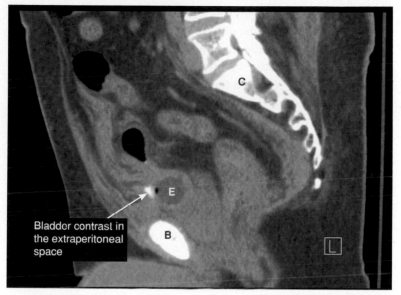

Bladder contrast in the extraperitoneal space

FIGURE 12.27 E

Pelvic Fractures

- Pubic rami fractures
  - Associated with sacral fractures
  - Stable fracture
- Pelvic ring fractures
  - High-energy trauma
  - Vertical fracture through posterior pelvis or sacrum: "open book" fracture
  - Associated with bladder, ureter, urethral, and kidney injuries
  - Unstable fracture

RADIOLOGY

- **Plain film findings** (Fig. 12.28)
  - Unstable injuries are defined by injuries in the anterior and posterior aspects of the pelvic ring
  - Lateral compressive forces usually result in fractures of the superior and inferior pubic rami as well as a unilateral fracture of the sacral ala

- Anteroposterior compressive forces result in widening of the sacroiliac joints and the pubic symphysis
- Vertical shear forces result in fracture of the ilium or sacrum as well as the superior and inferior rami
- Straddle injury results in fractures of the ischii and pubic rami
- Fractures of the sacrum and coccyx are usually from a fall on the buttocks and are best diagnosed on coned-down lateral views
- Avulsion injuries are due to muscles causing a fragment of the bone to be broken off its parent bone
- Insufficiency fractures of the elderly are common in the sacral ala seen best with MRI or scintigraphy
- Acetabular fractures are sometimes associated with dislocation of the femoral head
- **CT findings** (Fig. 12.29)
  - More precise method of evaluating injuries
- **Scintigraphy findings**
  - Helpful for diagnosing insufficiency fractures of the sacral ala
  - Honda sign = configuration of increased activity in the shape of the letter "H" representing bilateral sacral insufficiency fractures

FIGURE 12.28 A–D

FIGURE 12.28 A

A. Minimally displaced fracture of the superior right pubic ramus
B. Sacrum
C. Ilium
D. Ischium
E. Left pubic bone
F. Acetabulum
G. Femoral head
H. Greater trochanter
I. Lesser trochanter
J. Femur

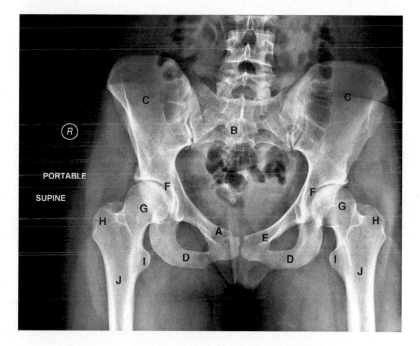

FIGURE 12.28 B

A. Diastasis of pubic symphysis   D. Pubic bone
B. Left sacral fracture   E. Acetabulum
C. Ischium

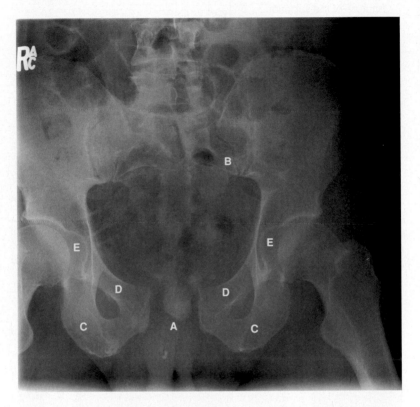

FIGURE 12.28 C

A. Left acetabular fracture
B. Left inferior pubic ramus fracture
C. Femoral head

D. Sacrum
E. Femoral shaft

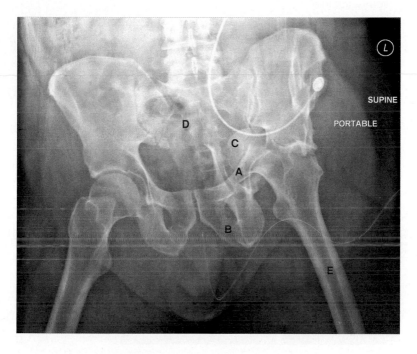

FIGURE 12.28 D

A. Right superior pubic ramus fracture

B. Right inferior pubic ramus fracture

C. Acetabulum

D. Femoral head

E. Sacrum

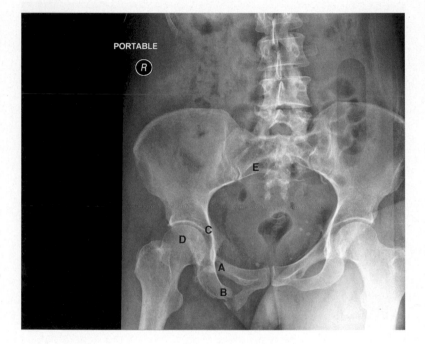

FIGURE 12.29 A-E

FIGURE 12.29 A

A. Right iliac fracture   C. Sacrum
B. Sacroiliac joint   D. Ilium

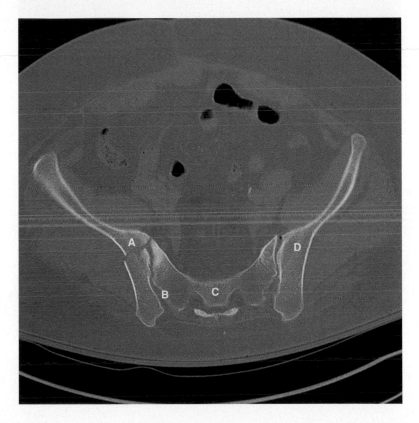

FIGURE 12.29 B

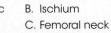

A. Right superior pubic ramus fracture

B. Ischium

C. Femoral neck

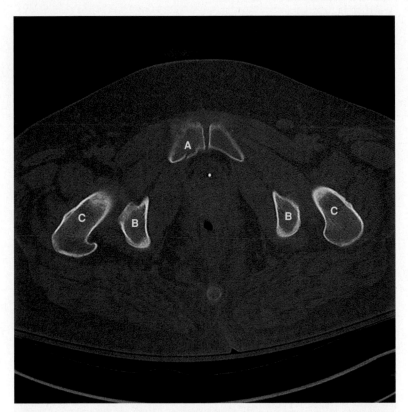

FIGURE 12.29 C

A. Right inferior pubic ramus fracture
B. Femur

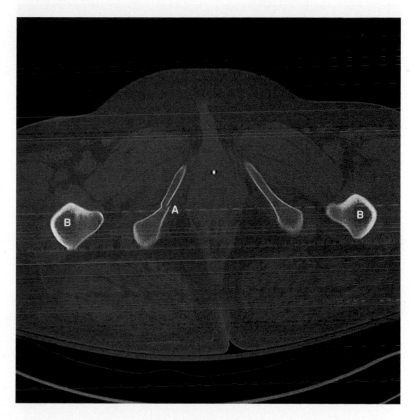

FIGURE 12.29 D

A. Right iliac fracture   C. Femur
B. Ischium   D. Sacrum

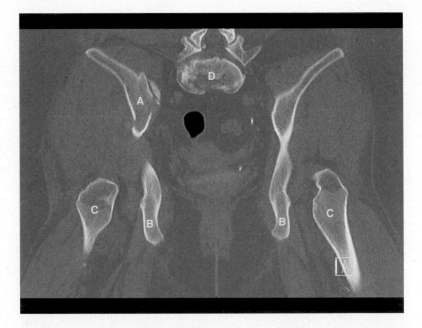

FIGURE 12.29 E

A. Iliac fracture
B. Acetabulum
C. Femoral head

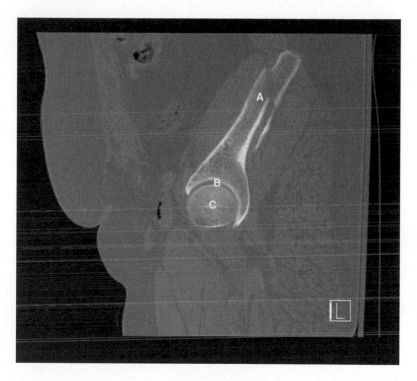

Suggested Readings

Brunicardi FC, Schwartz SI. *"Trauma." Schwartz's Principles of Surgery.* New York, NY: McGraw-Hill, Health Pub. Division, 2005.

Kaewlai R, Avery L, Asrani A, et al. Multidetector CT of blunt thoracic trauma. *Radiographics.* 2008;28:1555–1570.

Koo A, LaRoque R. Evaluation of head trauma by computed tomography. *Radiology.* 1977;123:345–350.

Nunez D, Zuluaga A, Fuentes-Bernardo D, et al. Cervical spine trauma: How much more do we learn by routinely using helical CT? *Radiographics.* 1996;16: 1307–1318.

Roberts J, Dalen K, Bosanko C, et al. CT in abdominal and pelvic trauma. *Radiographics.* 1993;13:735–752.

Sabiston DC, Townsend CM. *"Trauma." Sabiston Textbook of Surgery: The Biological Basis of Modern Surgical Practice.* Philadelphia, PA: Saunders/Elsevier; 2008.

Soto J, Anderson S. Multidetector CT of blunt abdominal trauma. *Radiology.* 2012;265:678–693.

Wilmore DW. *"Trauma." ACS Surgery: Principles and Practice.* New York, NY: WebMD; 2002.

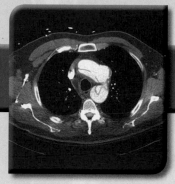

Vascular

Abdominal Aortic Aneurysm (AAA)

Overview

- Defined as >50% dilation of the vessel's normal size
- 90% AAAs are infrarenal
- Average growth of 3 to 4 mm/yr
- Rupture risk directly related to size (Laplace's law)
- Most are a result of atherosclerotic disease

Normal Vessel Dimensions

- Infrarenal aorta, 1.8 to 3 cm
- Common iliac, 0.8 to 1.6 cm
- External iliac, 0.6 to 1 cm

Signs and Symptoms

- Most found incidentally on imaging
- Physical examination is neither sensitive nor specific for asymptomatic aneurysm
  - Possible findings include pulsatile abdominal mass
- Rupture or impending rupture
  - Back/abdominal pain + pulsatile abdominal mass = AAA until proven otherwise
  - Hypotension/hypovolemic shock

Treatment/Management

- Elective repair if:
  - Men >5.5 cm, women >4.5 cm
  - Expansion >0.5 cm/6 mo

Size	Annual Rupture Risk	Estimated 5-year Rupture Risk
4–5 cm	1%	5–10%
5–6 cm	2–5%	30–40%
6–7 cm	3–10%	>50%
>7 cm	>10%	Up to 100%

- If not indicated for elective repair, follow up with CT scan or U/S every 6 months

RADIOLOGY

- While ultrasound is able to diagnose abdominal aortic aneurysms, CT is more able to define size, involvement of visceral arteries/renal arteries

Abdominal Aortic Aneurysm (AAA)

- **CT Findings** (Fig. 13.1)
  - The aneurysm can extend from below the level of the renal arteries to above the aortic bifurcation
  - May see mural thrombus

FIGURE 13.1 A–C

A. Kidney

B. Pulmonary hilum

C. Heart

D. Superficial femoral artery

E. Psoas muscle

F. Small bowel

G. Vertebra

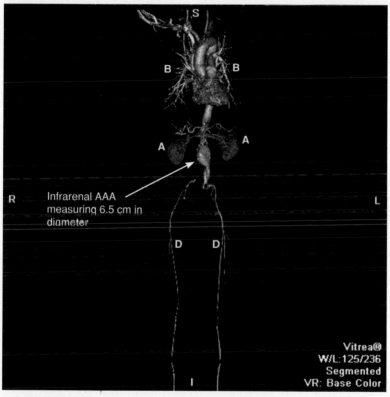

FIGURE 13.1 A

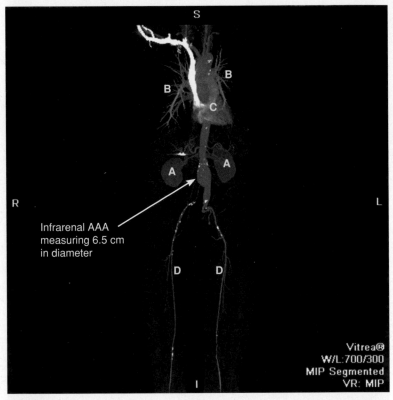

Infrarenal AAA measuring 6.5 cm in diameter

FIGURE 13.1 B

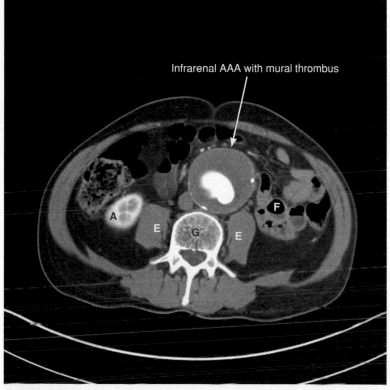

FIGURE 13.1 C

Descending Aortic Aneurysm with Rupture

- **CT findings** (Fig. 13.2)
  - Contrast extravasation from the aorta
  - Hemothorax due to blood collecting at the posterior aspects of the lung

FIGURE 13.2 A,B

A. Pulmonary vein	E. Main bronchus
B. Ascending aorta	F. Vertebra
C. SVC	G. Liver
D. Pulmonary artery	H. Kidney

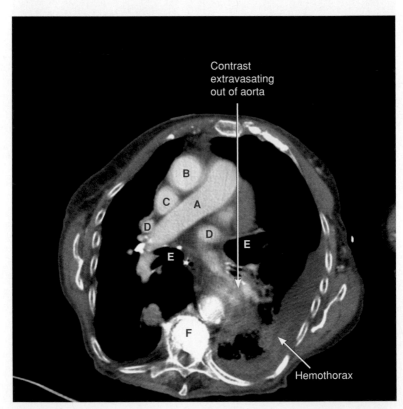

FIGURE 13.2 A

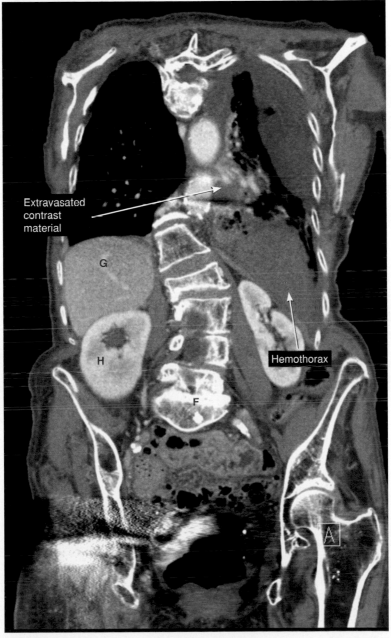

Extravasated
contrast
material

G

H

F

Hemothorax

FIGURE 13.2 B

Thoracic Aortic Aneurysm

Overview

- Defined as >50% dilation of the normal diameter
- Managed on the basis of location (ascending vs. arch vs. descending vs. thoracoabdominal)
- True aneurysm (involves all three layers of the arterial wall)
  - Saccular (localized outpouching) versus fusiform (more common)
- False aneurysm
  - Tear in vasa vasorum with bleeding into media layer
- Average expansion rate: Ascending aneurysm 0.7 mm/yr, descending 1.9 mm/yr

Etiology

- Nonspecific medial degeneration (result of imbalances between proteolytic enzymes); the most common cause
- Aortic dissection
- Genetic disorders: Marfan syndrome, Ehlers–Danlos syndrome, Loeys–Dietz syndrome, familial aortic aneurysmal disease
- Congenital bicuspid aortic valve
- Infectious: *Syphilis, Salmonella, Staphylococcus aureus, Staphylococcus epidermidis*
- Aortitis (chronic inflammation)

Signs and Symptoms

- Typically found incidentally
- May cause localized compression leading to chest pain
- Hoarseness with stretch of left recurrent laryngeal nerve
- High output heart failure with erosion into SVC
- Distal embolization
- Symptoms of rupture: Sudden severe chest pain (ascending), back pain (descending), flank and abdominal pain (thoracoabdominal), cardiac tamponade with rupture into pericardium

Treatment

- Medical management
  - Risk factor reduction (tobacco, hypercholesterolemia, hypertension)
  - Blood pressure control
  - Screen for other aneurysms since they are often associated with thoracic aortic aneurysm
- Open or endovascular surgical repair if:
  - Ascending >5.5 cm
  - Descending >6.5 cm
  - Repair at 5 cm if concurrent aortic valve replacement or 4.5 cm if undergoing bicuspid aortic valve replacement
  - Consider repair at 4 cm if it is associated with aortic regurgitation

RADIOLOGY

- **CXR**
  - Ascending: Convex shadow right of the cardiac silhouette, loss of the retrosternal space in the lateral view
  - Descending: Widening of descending aortic shadow, wall calcifications

Ascending Thoracic Aortic Aneurysm with Dissection (Fig. 13.3)

- **CT findings** (Fig. 13.3)
  - Dissection flap can extend from the aortic root up to the level of the right brachiocephalic artery
  - Blood surrounding the ascending aorta
  - Fat stranding noted in the pretracheal and aortopulmonary window fat
  - Aortic arch vessels are usually fed by the true lumen

FIGURE 13.3 A,B

A. Trachea
B. Sternum
C. Vertebra
D. Brachiocephalic artery

E. Left common carotid artery
F. Left subclavian artery
G. Aortic arch

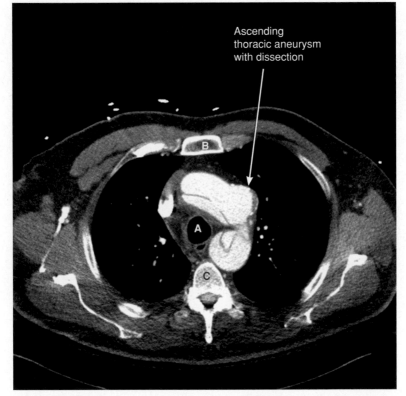

Ascending thoracic aneurysm with dissection

FIGURE 13.3 A

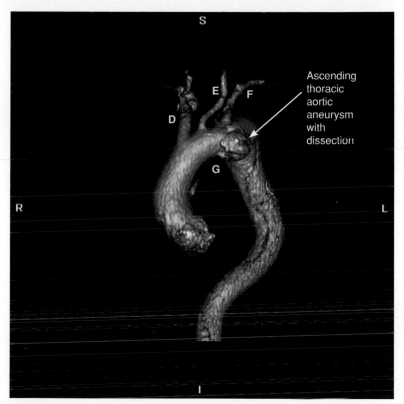

Ascending
thoracic
aortic
aneurysm
with
dissection

FIGURE 13.3 B

Descending Thoracic Aortic Aneurysm

- **Plain film findings** (Fig. 13.4)
  - Convexity of the descending aortic stripe, sometimes with wall calcifications
- **CT findings** (Fig. 13.4)
  - Thoracic aorta diameter exceeding 4 cm is considered aneurysmal
  - Can be associated with mural thrombus

FIGURE 13.4 A–C

A. Vertebra
B. Main bronchus
C. Left ventricle

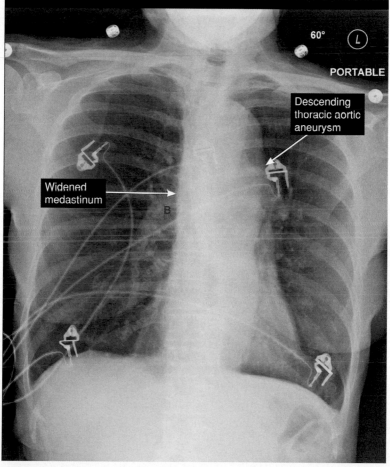

FIGURE 13.4 A

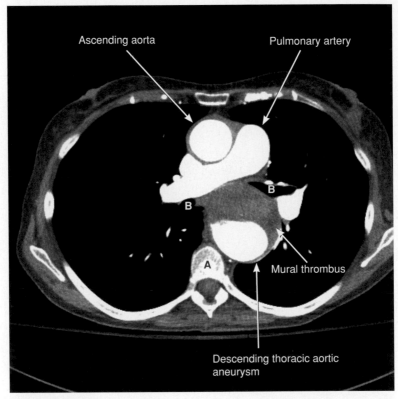

FIGURE 13.4 B

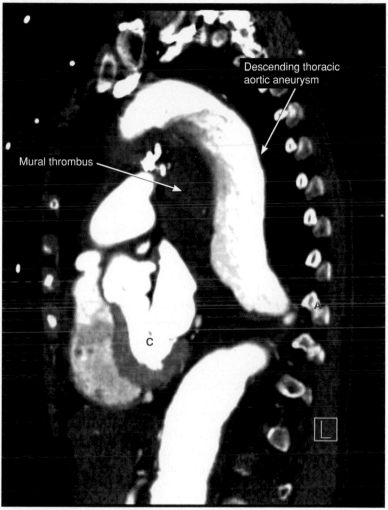

FIGURE 13.4 C

Aortic Dissection

Overview

- Tear in the intima layer resulting in the formation of two channels
  - True lumen
    - Lined by intima
  - False lumen
    - Within media
    - May compress true lumen causing malperfusion of aortic branches
    - Prone to rupture
- Risk factors
  - Smoking, HTN, HLP, atherosclerosis
  - Connective tissue disorders, aortitis, bicuspid aortic valve
  - Iatrogenic injury during cardiac catheterization
  - Drug use (cocaine)
- Classification:
  - Stanford Type A: Ascending dissection
  - Stanford Type B: Descending dissection
- Acute (<14 days) versus chronic (>14 days) versus subacute (15 to 60 days)

Signs and Symptoms

- Severe chest and back pain, typically described as tearing in nature
- If extended into coronary arteries, may present with symptoms of MI
- May manifest via occlusion of other aortic branches (mesenteric ischemia, renal failure, lower limb ischemia, etc.)

Diagnosis

- CXR
  - 10% to 15% have a normal CXR
  - Widened mediastinum
- CT with contrast
  - Double lumen aorta
  - Can assess other vessel involvement and presence of sequelae such as infarction of organs
  - Sensitivity 98%, specificity 89%

- MRA
  - Can be performed without contrast to evaluate for dissection (helpful if the patient is in renal failure)

Treatment

- Antihypertensive therapy
  - Goal SBP 100 to 110 mm Hg
  - Goal MAP 60 to 75 mm Hg with maintained urine output
  - HR 60 to 80 bpm
- Ascending aortic dissection is a surgical emergency
- Descending aortic dissection
  - Medical management unless rupture, malperfusion
- Chronic dissection
  - Repeat CT in 6 weeks following onset, q3 months × 1 year, q6 months × 1 year, then yearly
  - More frequent if connective tissue disorder or rapid expansion

RADIOLOGY

Aortic Transection

- **Plain film findings** (Fig. 13.5)
  - Widened mediastinum
  - Indistinctness of aortic knob
  - Left sided pleural effusion
  - Left apical cap seen as an opacity in the apical region of the left lung
  - Inferior displacement of the left bronchus
  - Tracheal deviation to the right
- **CT findings** (Fig. 13.5)
  - High attenuation mediastinal fluid, representing blood
  - Aortic wall disruption at the location of transection
  - High attenuation pleural effusion, representing a hemothorax

FIGURE 13.5 A,B

A. Vertebra
B. Main bronchus
C. Clavicle

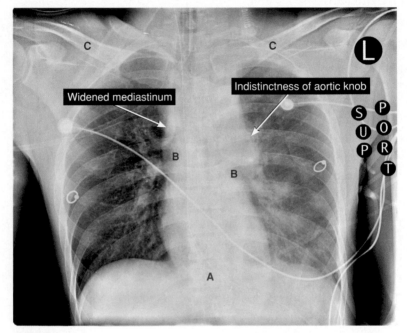

FIGURE 13.5 A

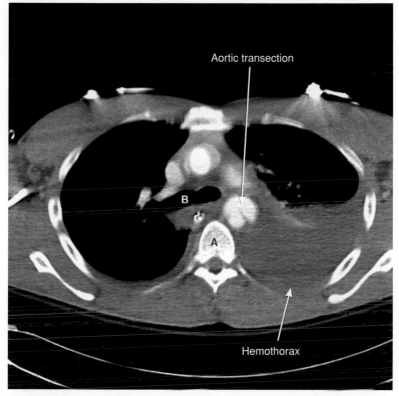

Aortic transection

B

A

Hemothorax

FIGURE 13.5 B

Aortic Dissection Type A (Fig. 13.6) and Type B (Fig. 13.7)

- **Plain film findings**
  - Mediastinal widening
  - Enlarged ascending aorta seen as a bulge to the right of the mediastinum above the right atrium shadow
  - Diffuse enlargement of the aorta
  - Pleural and pericardial effusions
- **CT findings** (Figs. 13.6 and 13.7)
  - Crescentic high-attenuating clot within the media of aortic wall best seen on noncontrast images
  - Intimal flap separating two aortic channels involving the ascending aorta
  - Hemothorax, hemopericardium, or hemomediastinum may be seen

FIGURE 13.6 A–C

A. Pulmonary artery
B. Pulmonary vein
C. Descending aorta
D. Superior vena cava

E. Vertebra
F. Left ventricle
G. Right atrium
H. Right ventricle

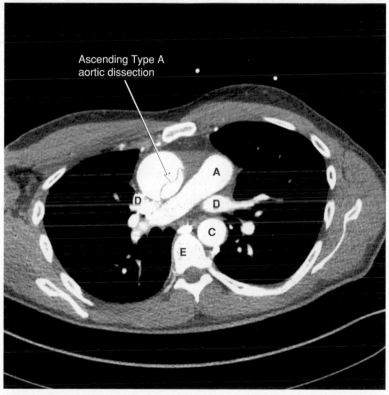

Ascending Type A aortic dissection

FIGURE 13.6 A

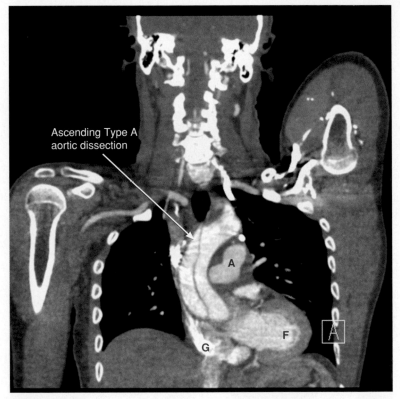

FIGURE 13.6 B

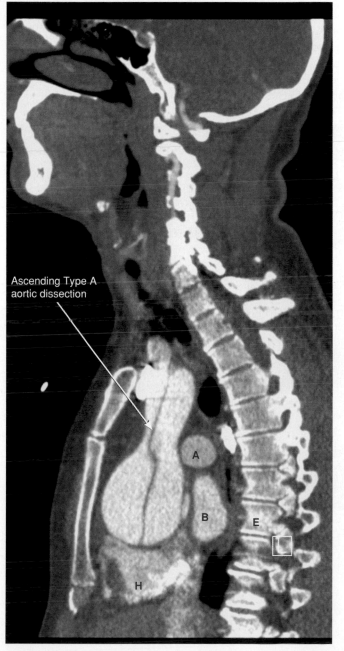

Ascending Type A
aortic dissection

FIGURE 13.6 C

FIGURE 13.7 A–C

A. Left ventricle
B. Right ventricle
C. Vertebra
D. Brachiocephalic artery
E. Left common carotid artery

F. Left subclavian artery
G. Celiac artery
H. Superior mesenteric artery
I. Renal artery
J. Common iliac artery

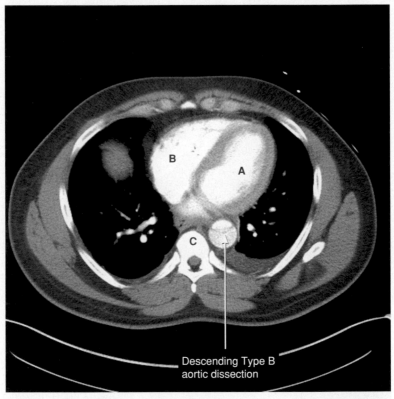

Descending Type B
aortic dissection

FIGURE 13.7 A

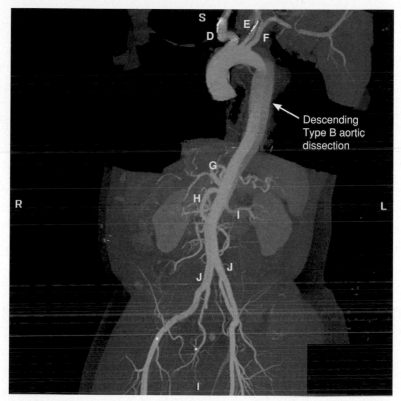

Descending Type B aortic dissection

FIGURE 13.7 B

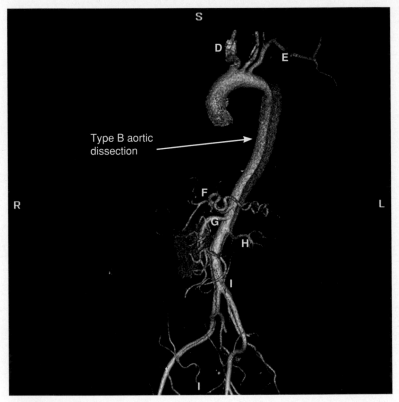

FIGURE 13.7 C

Iliac Artery Aneurysm (AAA)

Overview

- <2% of aneurysmal disease
- 10% to 20% of patients with AAA have iliac aneurysmal disease
- Typically presents in the seventh to eighth decade of life
- More common in men
- >70% common iliac, 20% internal iliac, rarely found in external iliac

Signs and Symptoms

- Vague lower abdominal pain/flank pain
- Compressive symptoms
  - Pyelonephritis, pain with defecation
  - Paresthesia of lower extremity
- May be palpated on physical examination when 4 cm or larger

Diagnosis

- Most of the time it is an incidental finding
- May be well visualized on ultrasound, CT, MRI, angiography

Treatment/Management

- Electively repaired if >3.5 cm
- Screen for AAA

RADIOLOGY

- **CT findings** (Fig. 13.8)
  - Diameter of the iliac artery measuring more than 1.5 times the normal diameter of the iliac artery
  - Extensive vascular calcifications and nonocclusive mural thrombus throughout the abdominal iliac trunk may be seen

FIGURE 13.8 A,B

A. Psoas muscle   D. Bladder
B. Vertebra   E. Cecum
C. Small bowel loops

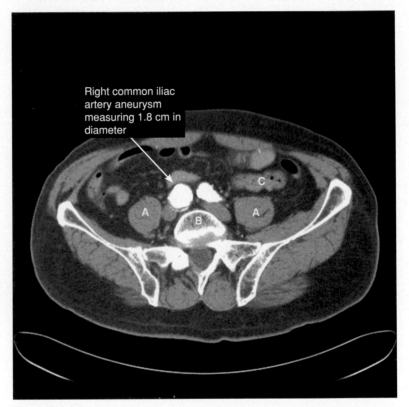

Right common iliac artery aneurysm measuring 1.8 cm in diameter

FIGURE 12.8 A

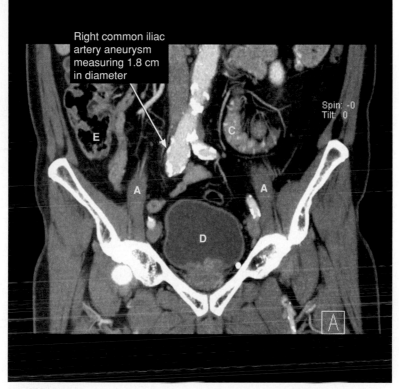

Right common iliac
artery aneurysm
measuring 1.8 cm
in diameter

Spin: -0
Tilt: 0

E

C

A

A

D

A

FIGURE 12.8 B

Popliteal Aneurysm

Overview

- Most common aneurysm in the periphery
- Often times found bilaterally
- Often times may have another aneurysm elsewhere

Signs and Symptoms

- Prominent popliteal pulses on examination
- May have claudication symptoms if there is a thrombus or emboli present

Diagnosis

- Most of the time it is an incidental finding
- May be well visualized on ultrasound, CT, MRI, and angiography

Treatment/Management

- Electively repair if >2 cm or if symptomatic
- Screen for AAA

RADIOLOGY

- **CT findings** (Fig. 13.9)
  - Aneurysm which occurs below the level of adductor hiatus and above the level of arterial bifurcation into anterior and tibioperoneal trunk arteries
  - Wall of aneurysm is thickened sometimes associated with perianeurysmal fat stranding
  - May be completely or partially thrombosed

FIGURE 13.9 A-D

A. Superficial femoral artery
B. Popliteal artery
C. Anterior tibial artery
D. Posterior tibial artery

E. Femur
F. Tibia
G. Patella
H. Fibula

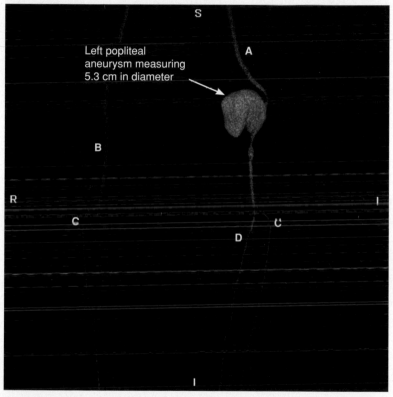

FIGURE 13.9 A

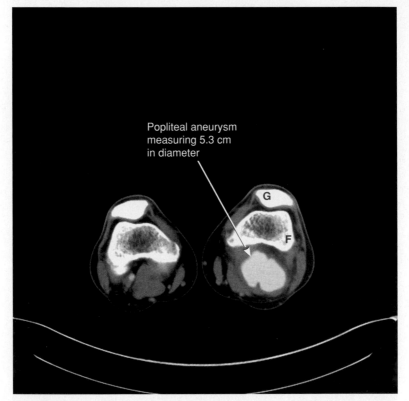

FIGURE 13.9 B

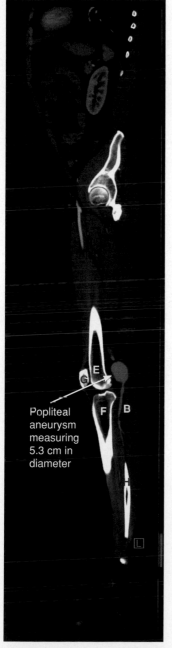

Popliteal aneurysm measuring 5.3 cm in diameter

FIGURE 13.9 C

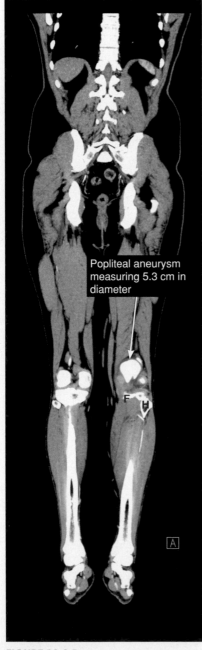

Popliteal aneurysm measuring 5.3 cm in diameter

FIGURE 13.9 D

Mycotic Aneurysm

Overview

- Infected aneurysm
- Rare (1% to 3% of aneurysms)
- Due to weakening of vessel wall by organism versus secondarily infected aneurysm
- Risk factors
  - Endocarditis
  - Atherosclerosis
  - Advanced age
  - Tobacco use
  - Immunosuppression
  - Drug users

Signs and Symptoms

- Nonspecific
- Fevers/chills, weight loss, malaise, sepsis
- Massive hemorrhage versus fulminant sepsis

Diagnosis

- Positive blood cultures in 50% to 75% of the time
- CT
  - New, focal aneurysm, sometimes with perivascular gas or fat stranding
- Ultrasound
  - Focal outpouching from the artery with surrounding inflammation

Treatment

- Antibiotics and surgery
  - Broad spectrum antibiotics for gram-positive and gram-negative coverage
  - Most commonly *Staphylococcus aureus,* Streptococci, Salmonella, Treponemal, Mycobacterial, fungal
  - Fifty percent mortality with medical therapy alone
  - Surgical intervention to confirm diagnosis, control source, prevent rupture
  - Potentially requires lifelong antibiotics without source control

RADIOLOGY

- **CT findings** (Fig. 13.10)
  - Focal outpouching of contrast arising from an artery
  - Soft tissue inflammation around a vessel
  - Sometimes associated with intramural air or air collection around the vessel
  - Perivascular fluid collection may be present

FIGURE 13.10 A–F

A. Descending aorta
B. Splenic artery
C. Hepatic artery
D. Superior mesenteric artery
E. Common iliac artery

F. Kidney
G. Inferior vena cava
H. Liver
I. Spleen

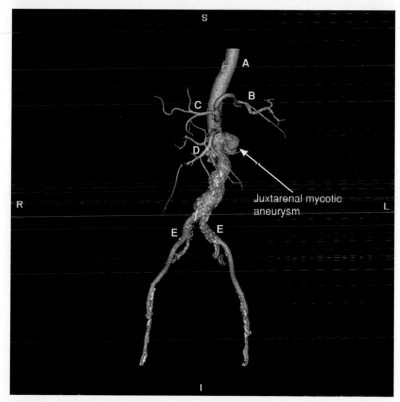

Juxtarenal myootic aneurysm

FIGURE 13.10 A

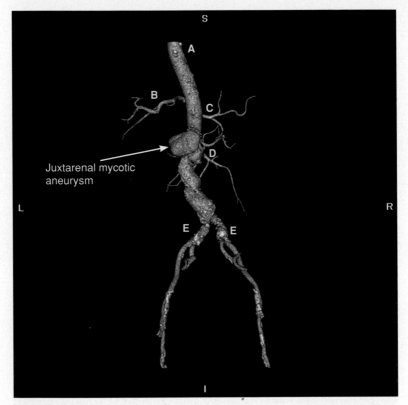

FIGURE 13.10 B

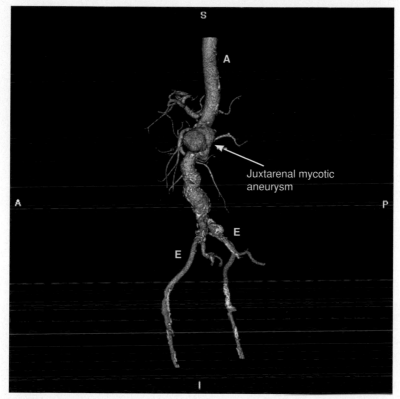

FIGURE 13.10 C

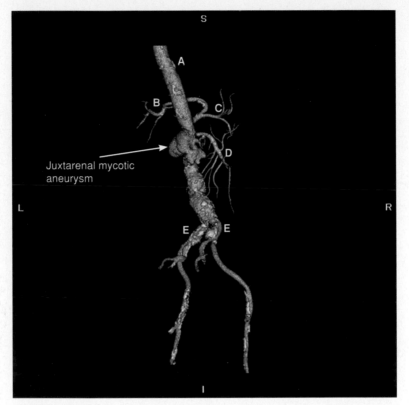

Juxtarenal mycotic aneurysm

FIGURE 13.10 D

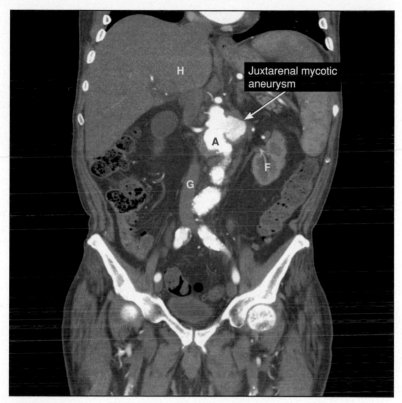

Juxtarenal mycotic aneurysm

FIGURE 13.10 E

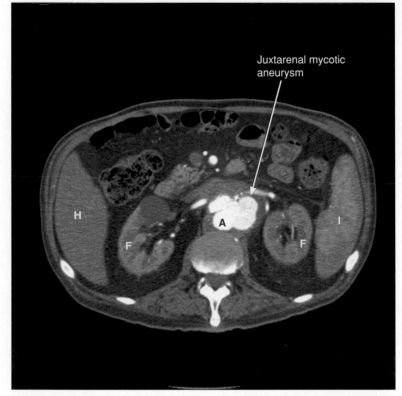

FIGURE 13.10 F

Aortoenteric Fistula

Overview

- Fistula typically between the third or fourth portion of duodenum and the aorta
- Usually secondary to aortic surgery
- Other causes include AAA rupture, perforated duodenal ulcer
- Mortality is 30% in recognized cases, 100% in unrecognized cases

Signs and Symptoms

- GI hemorrhage, pulsatile mass, and infection
- Herald bleed followed by massive hemorrhage (hours to days later)
- Half of the patients report abdominal or back pain initially

Imaging

- CT is test of choice

Treatment

- Resection with extra-anatomic bypass

RADIOLOGY

- **CT findings** (Fig. 13.11)
  - Periaortic air and surrounding fat stranding
  - Possible pseudoaneurysm
  - Fistulous connection between the aorta and bowel may be noted on contrast-enhanced scans as demonstrated by extravasation of contrast from the aorta into the bowel lumen
  - Possible extravasation of IV contrast within duodenal lumen or inner lumen of adjacent bowel walls

FIGURE 13.11 A,B

A. Liver
B. Gallbladder
C. Small bowel loops

D. Vertebra
E. Descending aorta

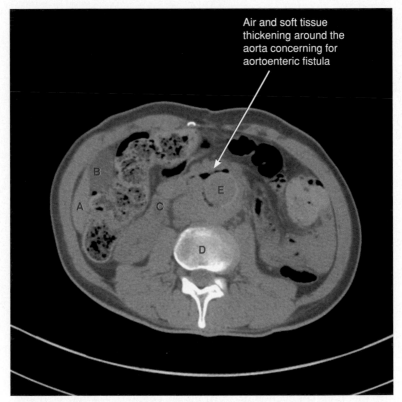

Air and soft tissue thickening around the aorta concerning for aortoenteric fistula

FIGURE 13.11 A

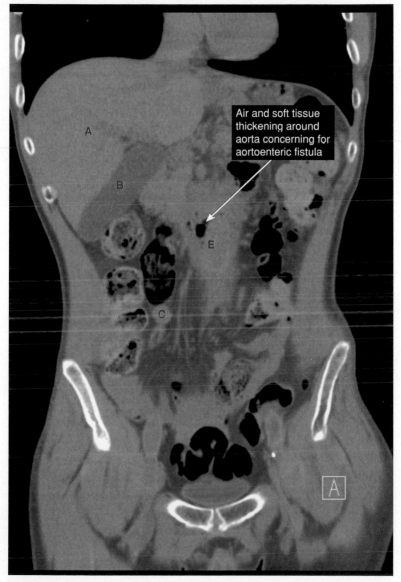

Air and soft tissue thickening around aorta concerning for aortoenteric fistula

FIGURE 13.11 B

Suggested Readings

Kayani I, Groves AM, Syed R. Aortoenteric fistula as shown by multidetector computed tomography. *Heart*. 2005;91:304.

Lee WK, Mossop PJ, Little AF, et al. Infected (mycotic) aneurysms: Spectrum of imaging appearances and management. *Radiographics*. 2008;28:1853–1868.

LePage MA, Quint LE, Sonnad SS, et al. Aortic dissection: CT features that distinguish true lumen from false lumen. *Am J Roentgenol*. 2001;177:207–211.

Marotta R, Franchetto AA. The CT appearance of aortic transection. *Am J Roentgenol*. 1996;166:647–651.

Orton DF, LeVeen RF, Saigh JA, et al. Aortic prosthetic graft infections: Radiologic manifestations and implications for management. *Radiographics*. 2000;20:977–993.

Rakita D, Newatia A, Hines JJ, et al. Spectrum of CT findings in rupture and impending rupture of abdominal aortic aneurysms. *Radiographics*. 2007;27:497–507.

Sakamoto I, Sueyoshi E, Hazama S, et al. Endovascular treatment of iliac artery aneurysms. *Radiographics*. 2005;25:S213–S227.

Sheth S, Fishman EK. Imaging of the inferior vena cava with MDCT. *Am J Roentgenol*. 2007;189:1243–1251.

Siegel CL, Cohan RH. CT of abdominal aortic aneurysms. *Am J Roentgenol*. 1994;163:17–29.

Wright LB, Matchett WJ, Cruz CP, et al. Popliteal artery disease: Diagnosis and treatment. *Radiographics*. 2004;24:467–479.

Index

Note: Page number followed by f indicates figure only.